Yoga and
Spiritual Retreats

The Deutsche Nationalbibliothek lists this publication in the Deutsche Nationalbibliografie; detailed bibliographic data are available on the Internet at http://dnb.dnb.de.

ISBN 978-3-03768-194-7
© 2015 by Braun Publishing AG
www.braun-publishing.ch

1st edition 2015

Editor: Sibylle Kramer
Editorial staff and layout: Maria Barrera del Amo
Translation: Geoffrey Steinherz
Graphic concept: Michaela Prinz, Berlin

Sibylle Kramer

Yoga and Spiritual Retreats

Relaxing Spaces to Find Oneself

BRAUN

Contents

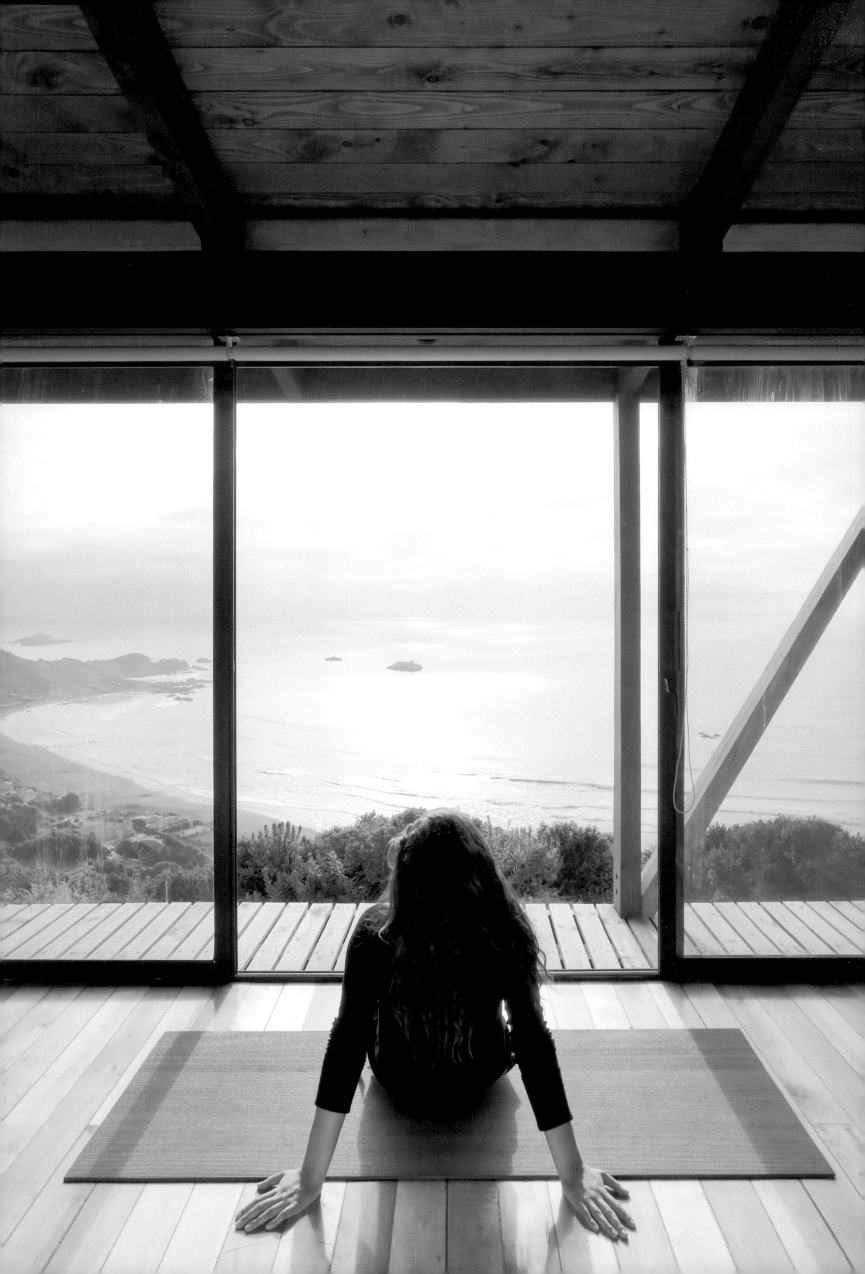

Preface

Yoga is one of the six classical schools of Indian philosophy, often described as a spiritual path in search
of enlightenment, as a connection between body, spirit
and soul. Or as a path to self-knowledge. Imagine the
individual as traveller in the material body, the coach. The
coachman is the understanding, the passenger is the soul
and the horses are the symbols for the five senses. Just
as the harness connects, yoga coordinates the individual
entities in a unity on the way to finding deliverance.

Asceticism and contemplation, concentration and meditation are important elements which can optimally develop
in an environment of quiet, a place of calm, retreat and
strength. This platform is ideally a built space that is in
conformity with the practice of yoga, merging with it in
a unity. The times have long since passed when there
were no alternatives to sweaty gymnasiums or badly lit,
soulless exercise rooms. Today, yoga rooms are designed
and staged with the attitude of their operators in mind:
as purist spaces clothed with complementarily unified
materials, which support the contemplation of one's own
consciousness, as an artistically arranged space which
offers inspiration and creativity. Or as a surreal location
for tuning out. Yoga rooms are design challenges which
follow the philosophy of their users. Sometimes it is the
physical training which is in the foreground, sometimes
the life style and the relaxation. Or the traditional, philo-
sophical point of view.

As varied and multifaceted as the architectural interpre-
tation of unity, integration and tension can be, it always
combines the revealed attitude and the rigorous realiza-
tion of the concept. For instance, the clearly structured
Yoga House by WMR architects places nature in the
foreground and integrates the building in the forceful
mountains' poetic surroundings. The *Yoga House* opens
itself up and bathes in nature. The room arrangement is
such that the landscape becomes part of a setting which
offers every guest a box seat. The function of the rooms
follows the progress of the sun, so that by force of nature
extraordinary conditions are created as an impetus for
concentration on what is most important. In a completely
different way the *KM Yoga Studio* by Tobias Partners
creates a similarly spiritual location. Wooden slats linearly
define the unity of the space, while translucent panels filter out a diffuse brightness from the daylight. The spatial
envelope repels all intrusions from the outside, creating
an intimate, self-reflective location for contemplation.

The approaches of the architects and designers are
manifold and well considered. Under the influence of the
location of nature and philosophy, unique spaces for the
mastering of body and spirit evolve, which on the way to
self-knowledge, contribute vigor, energy and inspiration.
So, sit back for a journey through some extraordinarily
designed places of quiet …

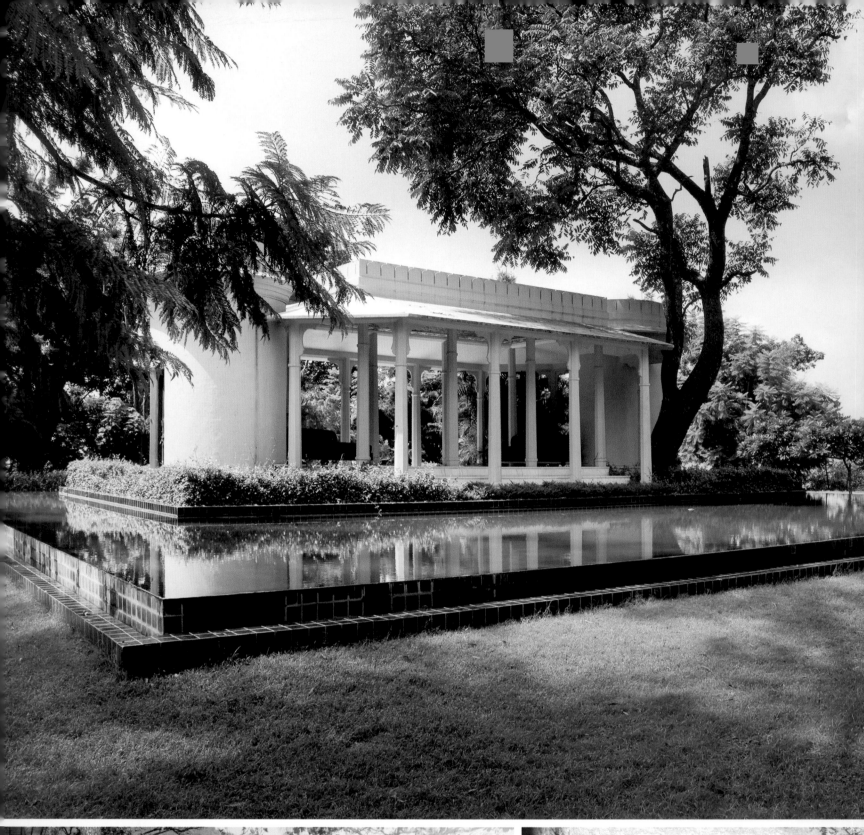

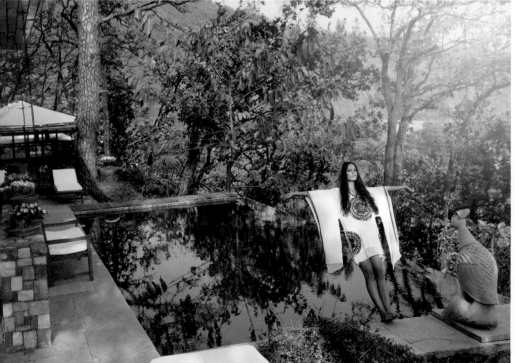

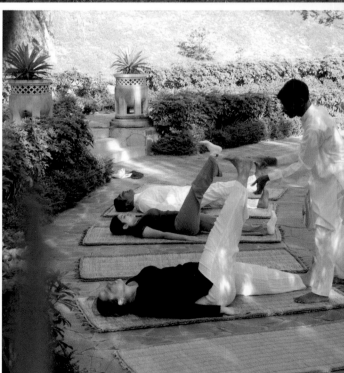

from above to below, from left to right: music pavilion for
meditation, villa-pool, morning group yoga at amphitheater

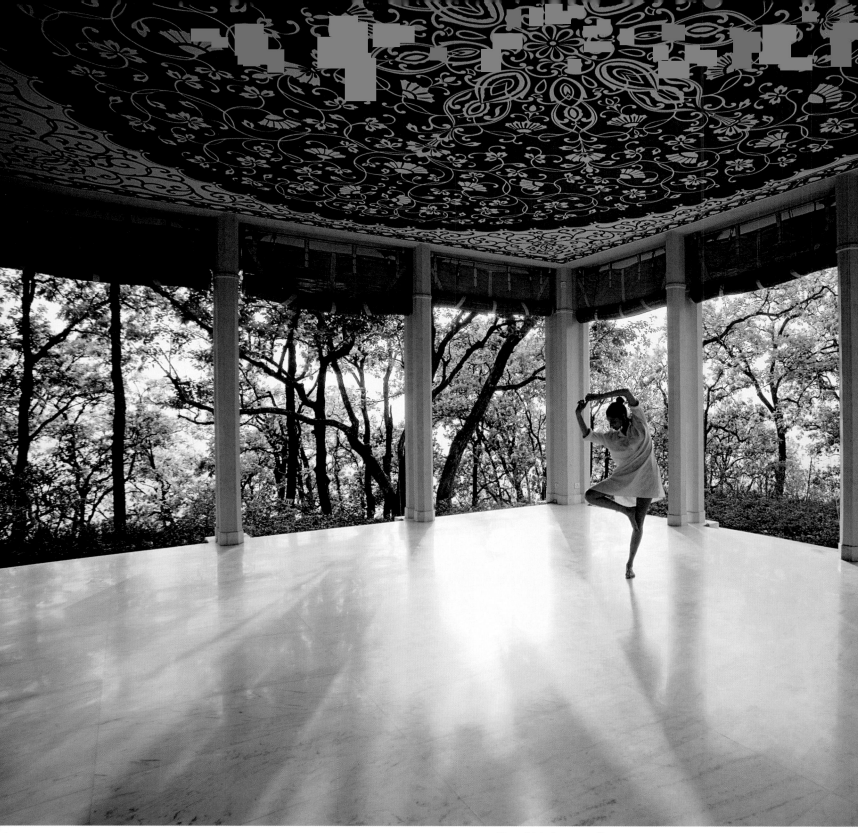

Hawa Mahal yoga pavilion

Ananda in the Himalayas

Uttarakhand, India

Architect: Chhada Siembieda & Associates
Location: The Palace Estate, Narendra Nagar, Tehri Garhwal, Uttarakhand, India
Year of completion: 2001
Type of retreat: health & wellness

Ananda is a multi-award winning luxury destination spa in the foothills of the majestic Himalayan Mountains. Overlooking the spiritual town of Rishikesh and the Ganges river valley in Northern India, Ananda is a retreat dedicated to restoring balance and harmonizing energy through a holistic approach to wellbeing. It integrates traditional Indian wellness practices of Ayurveda, yoga and vedanta with the best of international wellness experiences and healthy organic cuisine to bring about the union of mind, body and soul. The resort features exquisitely landscaped gardens, seventy elegant rooms with panoramic views, four suites with secluded private gardens, a historical presidential viceregal suite with its own private terrace and a rooftop jacuzzi and three private luxury villas, each with a private pool in the midst of Sal trees.

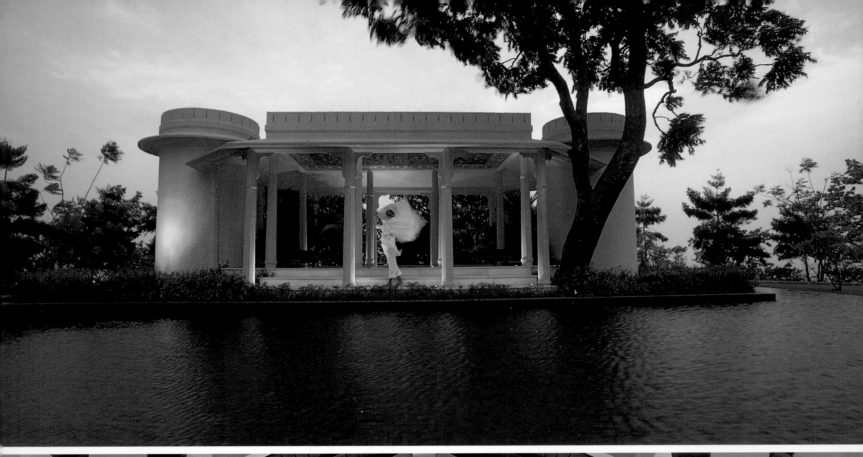

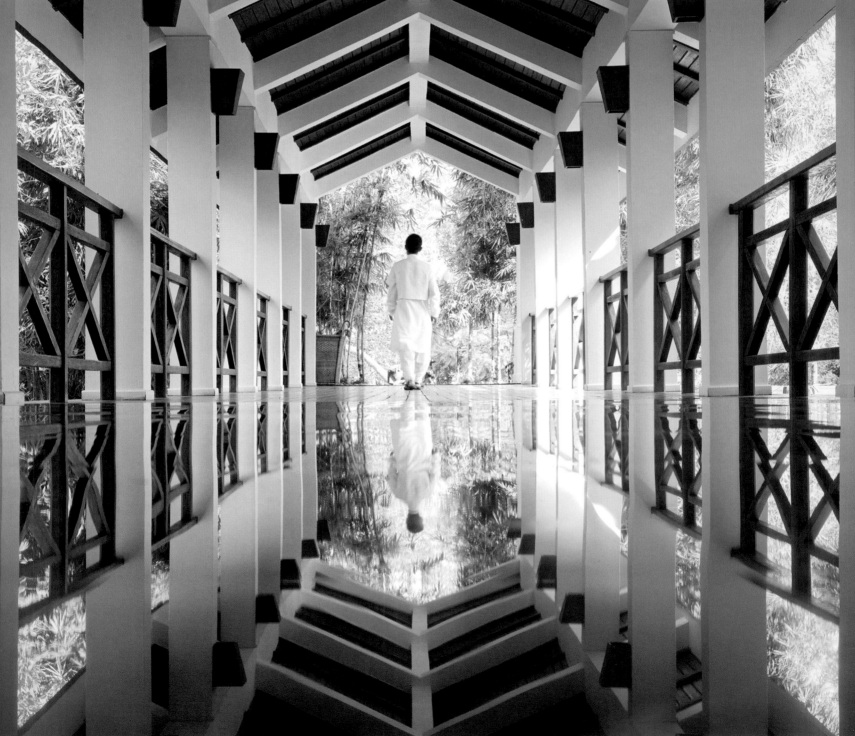

from above to below: yoga temple, hallway

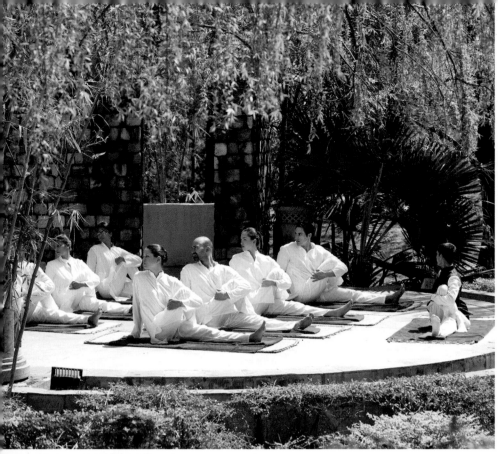

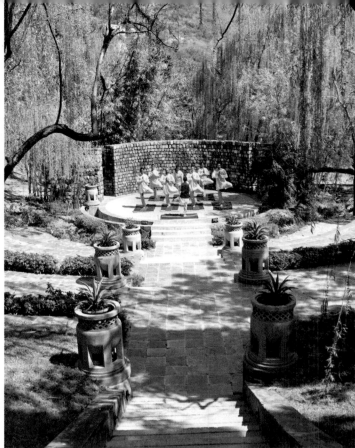

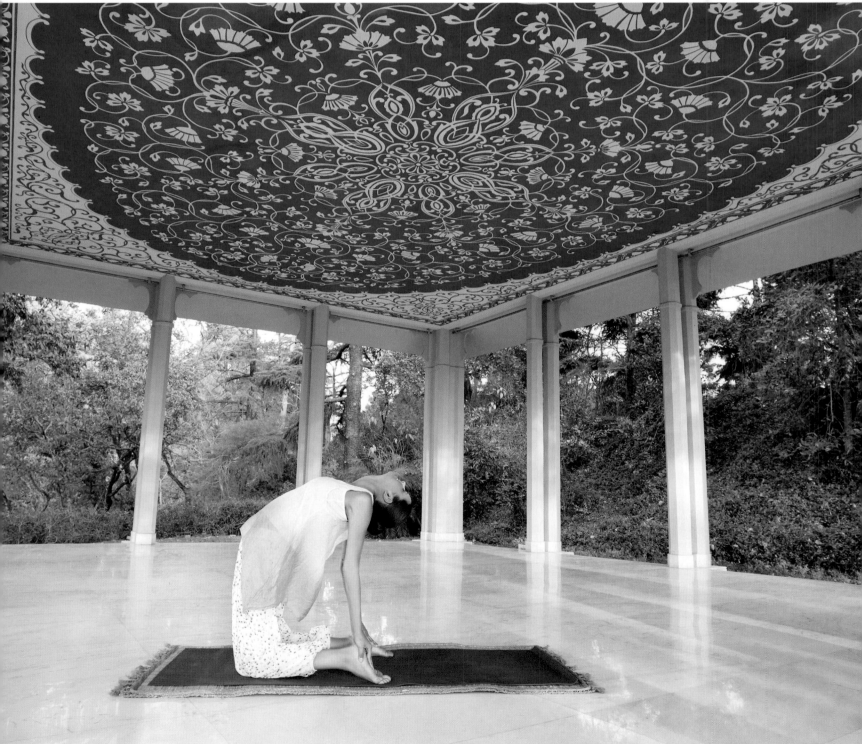

from above to below: yoga group, woman practicing yoga

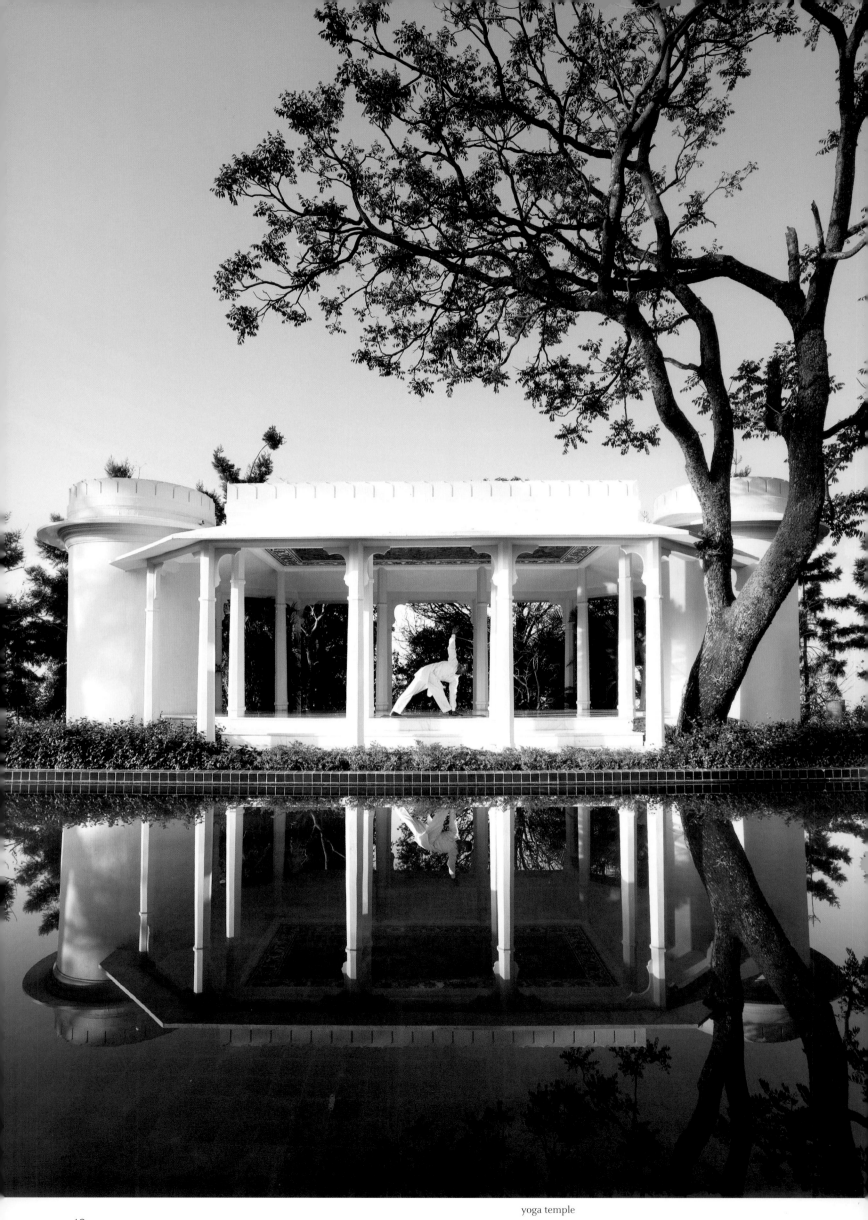

yoga temple

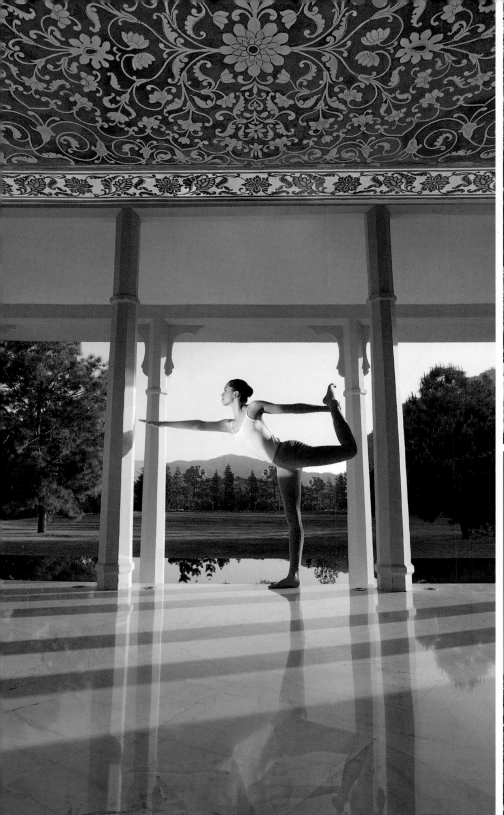

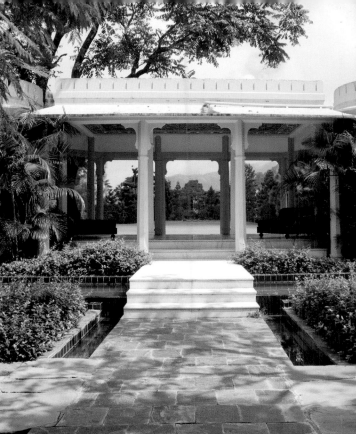

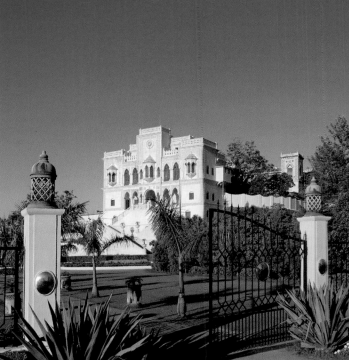

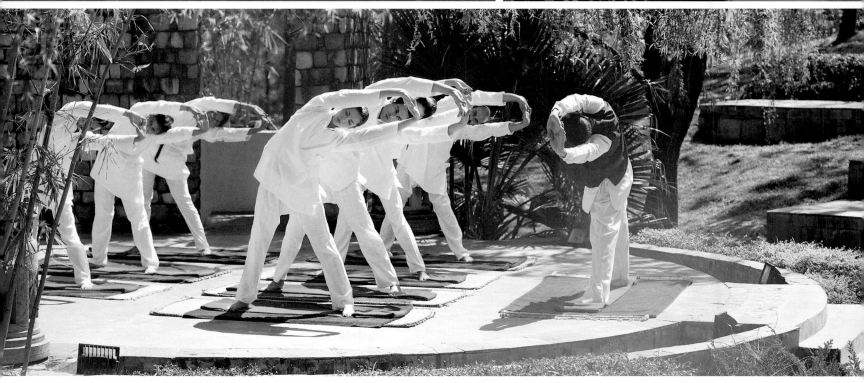

from left to right, from above to below: woman practicing
yoga, yoga temple, general view, people practicing yoga

13

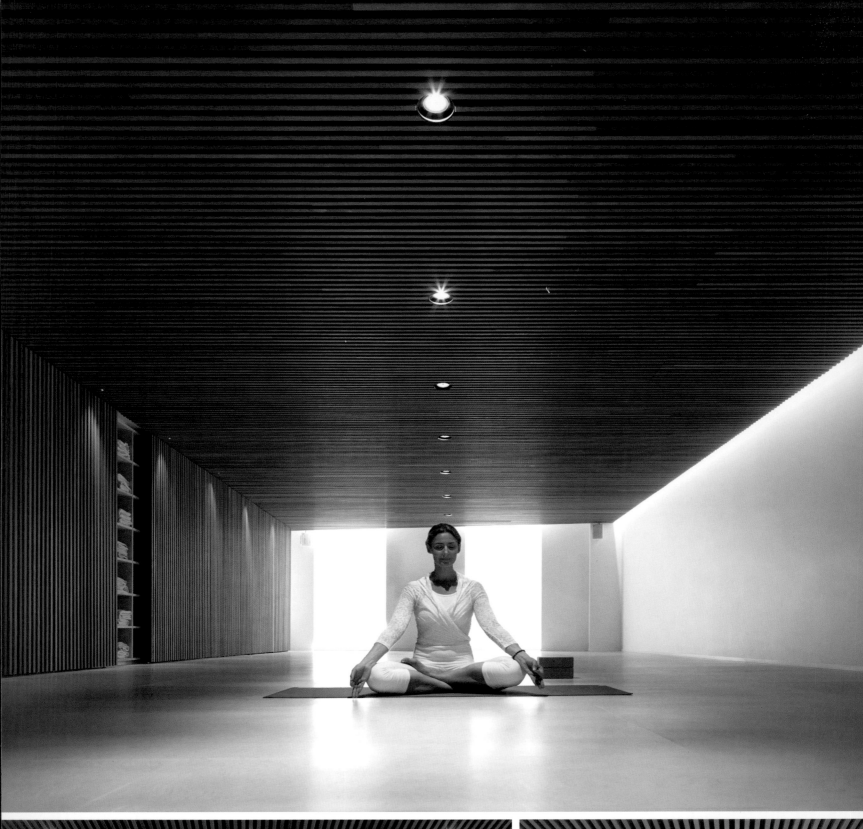

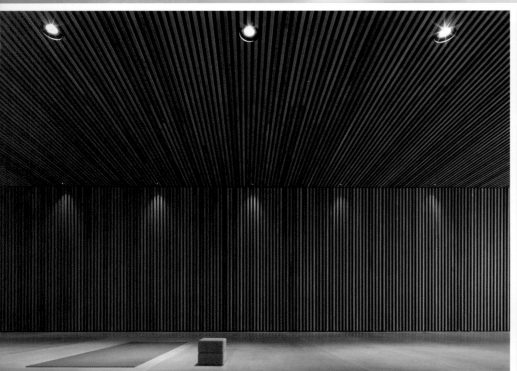

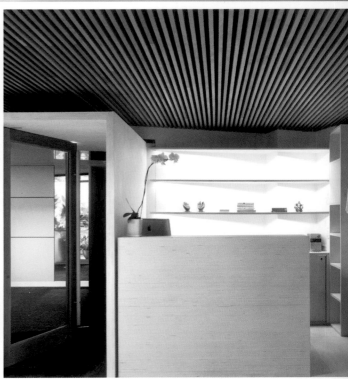

from above to below, from left to right: woman practicing yoga, yoga studio, reception

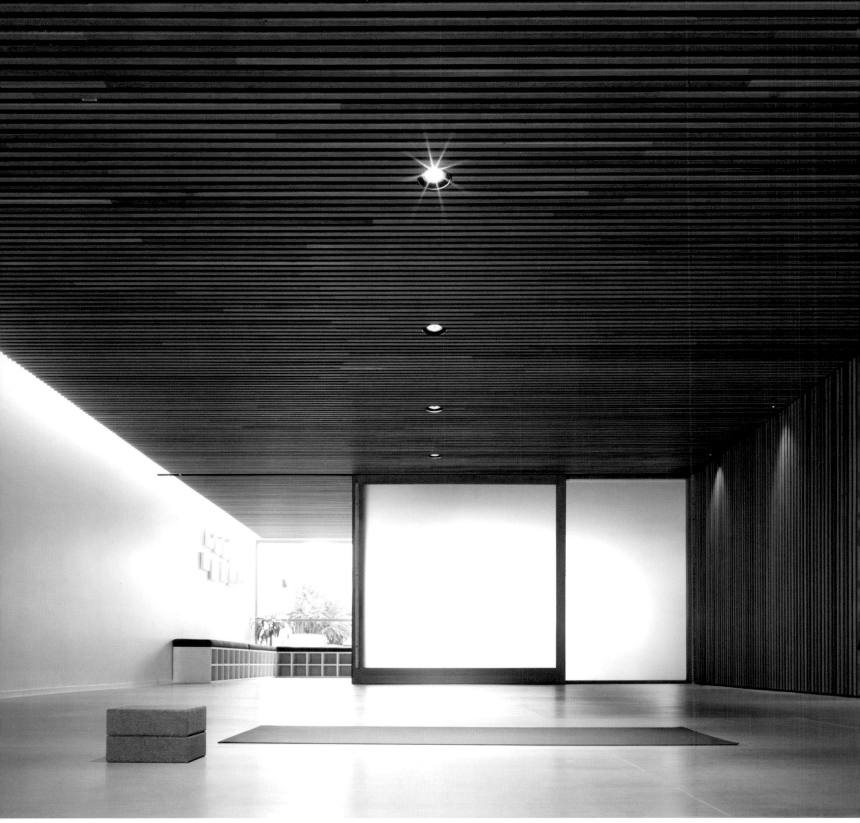

interior view

KM Yoga Studio

Bondi Junction, Australia

Architect:
Tobias Partners
Year of completion: 2012
Area: 116 sqm
Type of retreat: yoga studio

The brief for this yoga studio was to create an inspiring and peaceful place for the coming together of like-minded people. Through consistency of fabric and use of a singular natural material to line the walls and ceilings, a clear conceptual language resonates, defining the studio volume and its use. Intimate and nurturing, the space gently envelops the occupant, creating a serene experience.

Translucent screens diffuse the natural light, acting as a supple filter, while excluding any clear reference to or distractions from the outside world. The intent is to evoke a sense of total immersion. In its overall planning, its use of three-dimensional surfaces, and its detailing, KM Yoga is articulated as a space dedicated to, and at the same time evoking, strength and resolve.

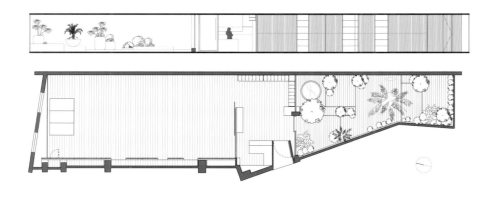

from above to below: section and floor plan, entrance

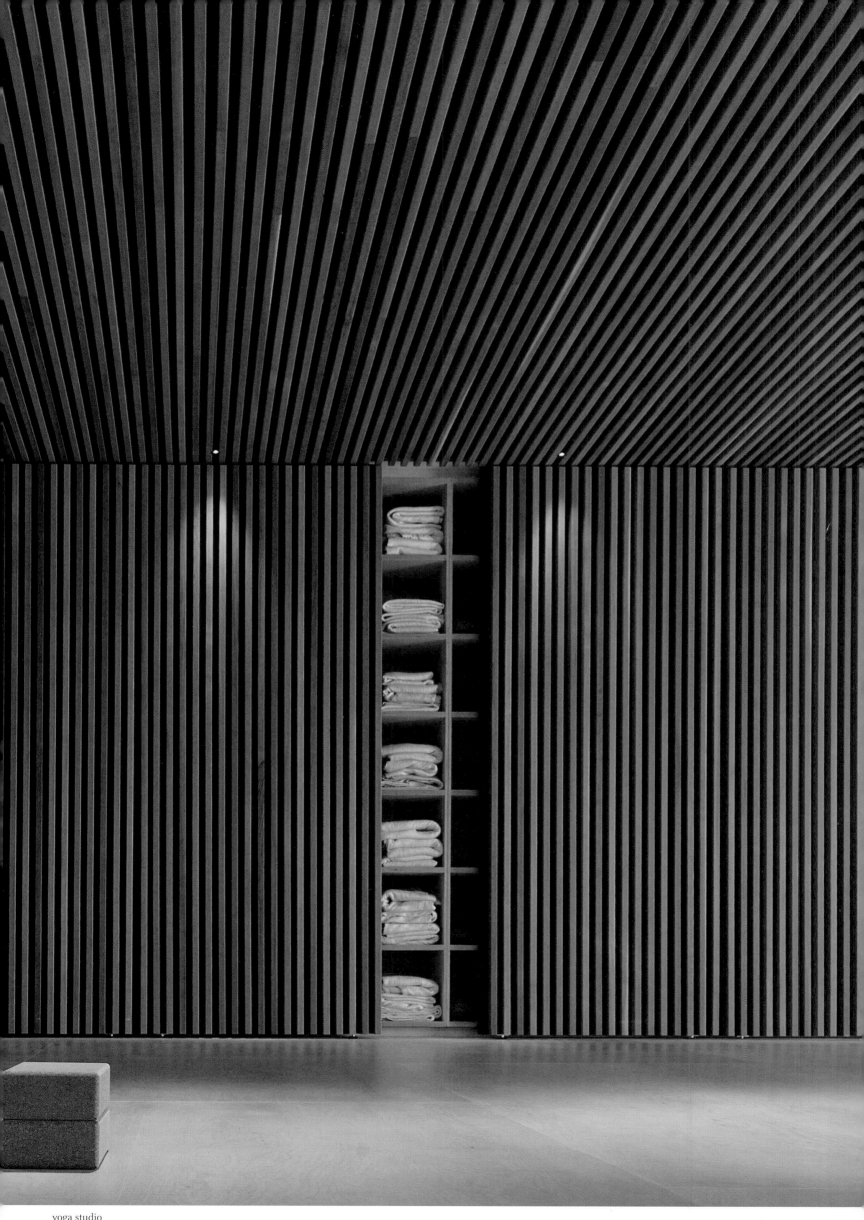

yoga studio

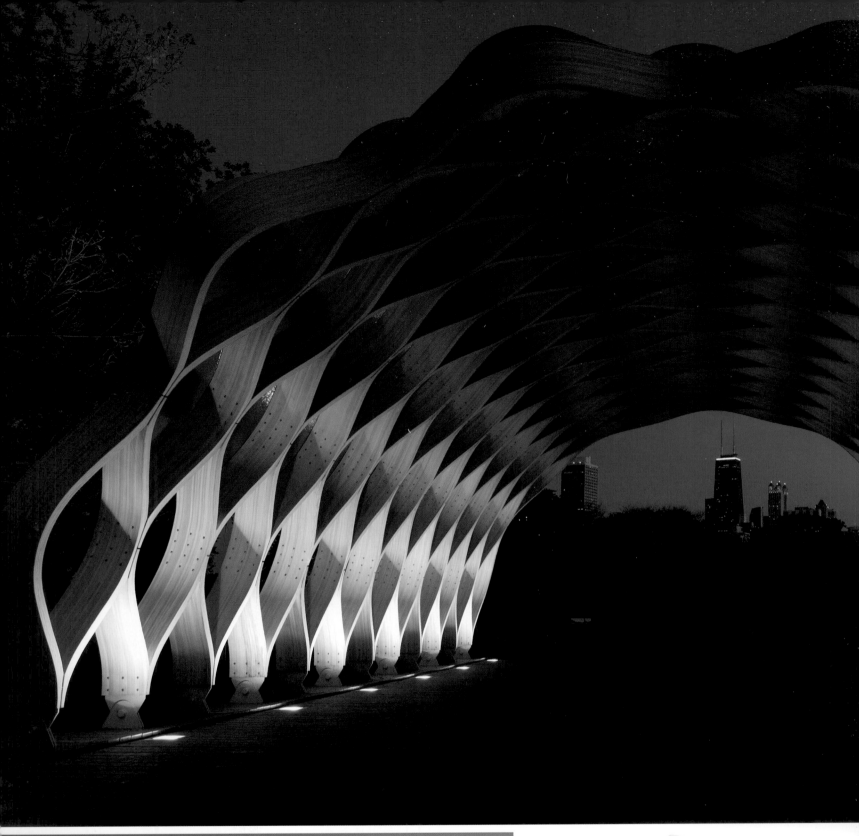

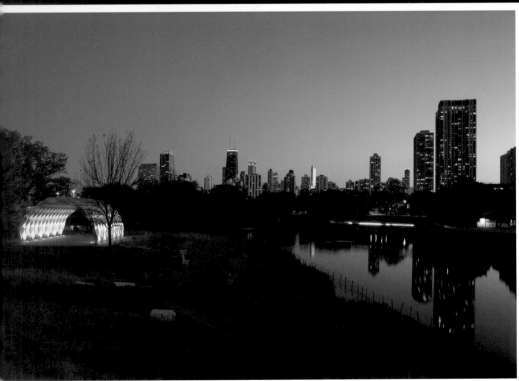

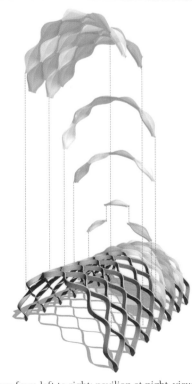

from above to below, from left to right: pavilion at night, view
with skyline, axonometric view

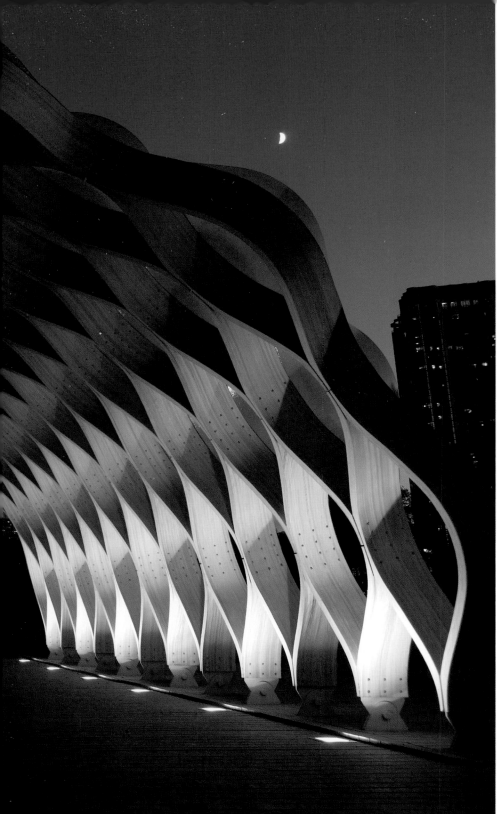

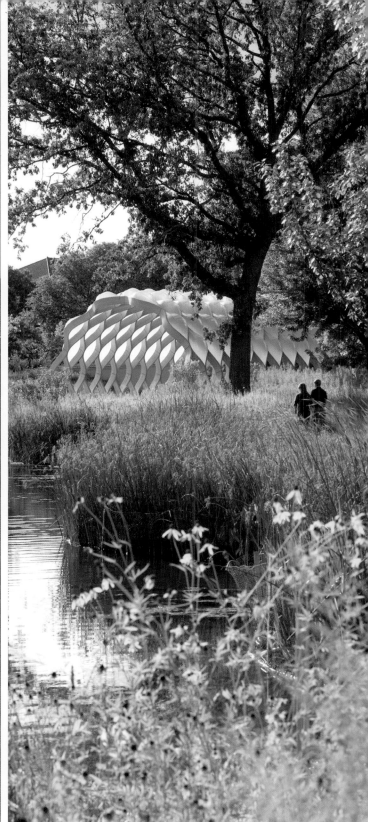

nature view

Nature Boardwalk

Chicago, USA

Architect: Studio Gang Architects
Location: Lincoln Park Zoo, Chicago, Illinois, USA
Year of completion: 2010
Type of retreat: pavilion and boardwalk on the zoo's south end

The project transforms a picturesque urban pond from the 19th century into an ecological habitat buzzing with life. With the design's improvements to water quality, hydrology, landscape, and accessibility, the site is able to function as an outdoor classroom in which the co-existence of natural and urban surroundings is demonstrated. A new boardwalk circumscribing the pond passes through various educational zones that explicate the different animals, plants, and habitat found in each. A pavilion integrated into the boardwalk sequence provides shelter for open-air yoga classes on the site. Inspired by the tortoise shell, its laminated structure consists of prefabricated, bent-wood members and a series of interconnected fiberglass pods that give global curvature to the surface.

19

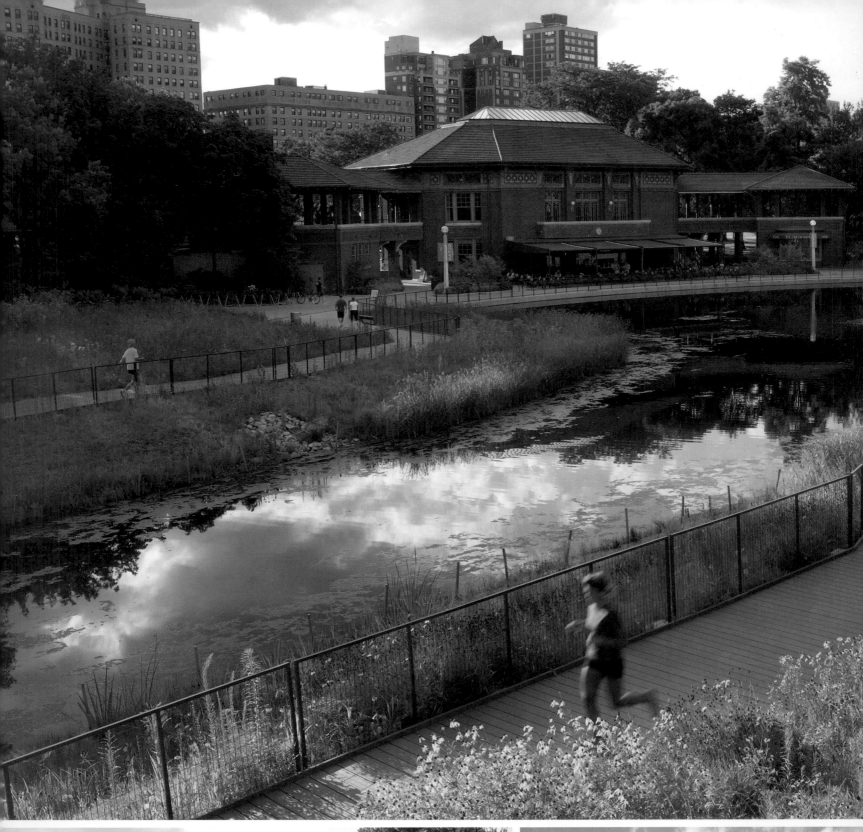

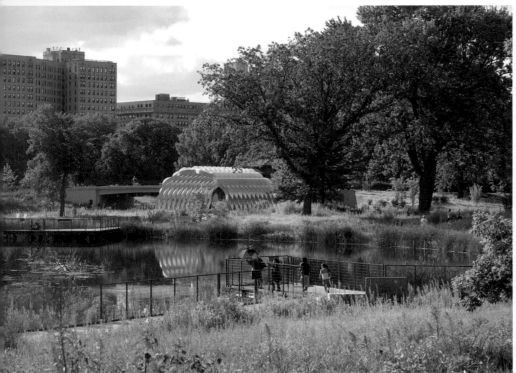

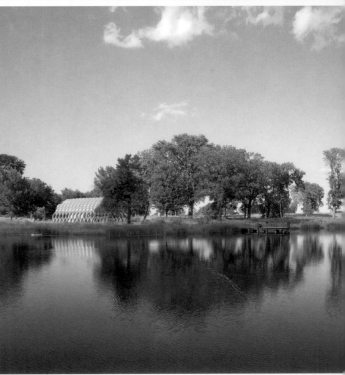

from above to below, from left to right: jogging path, general
view, pond view

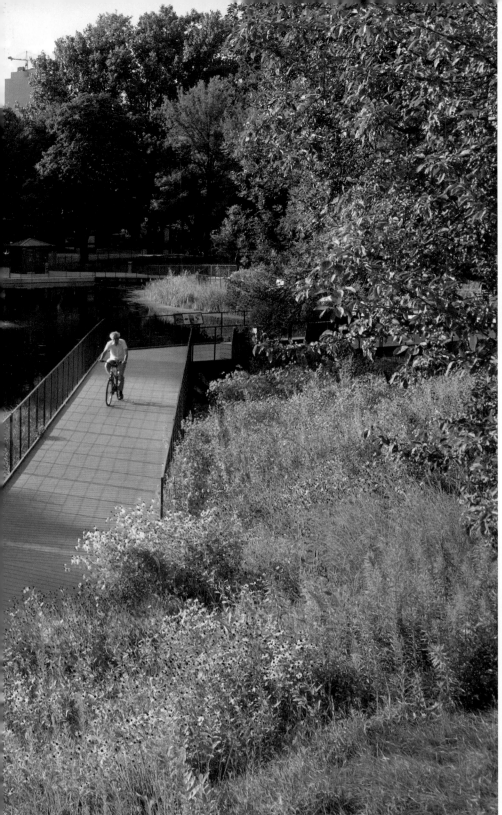

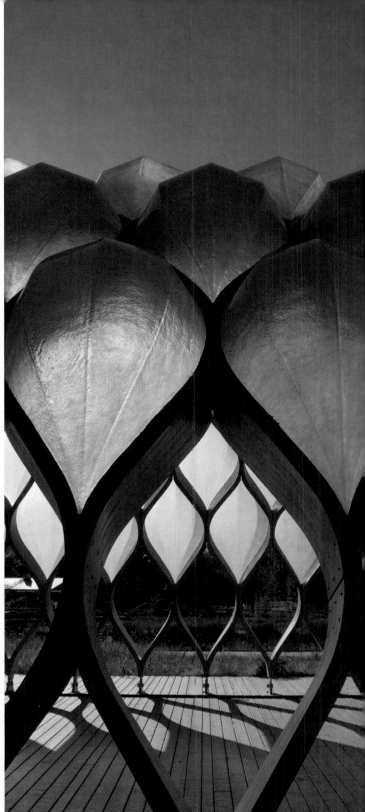

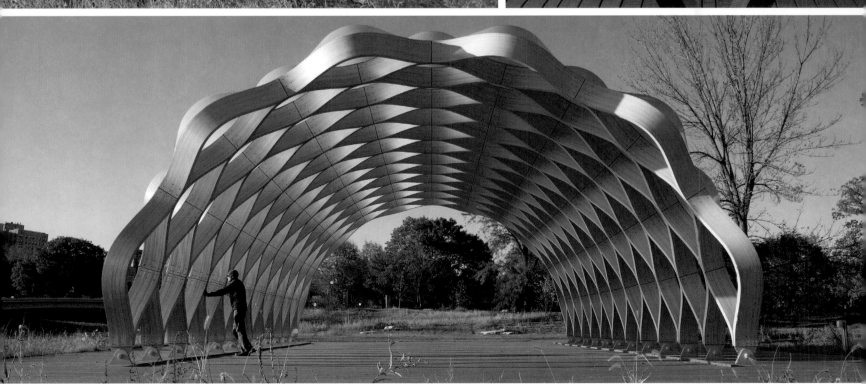

from above to below: detail, pavilion view

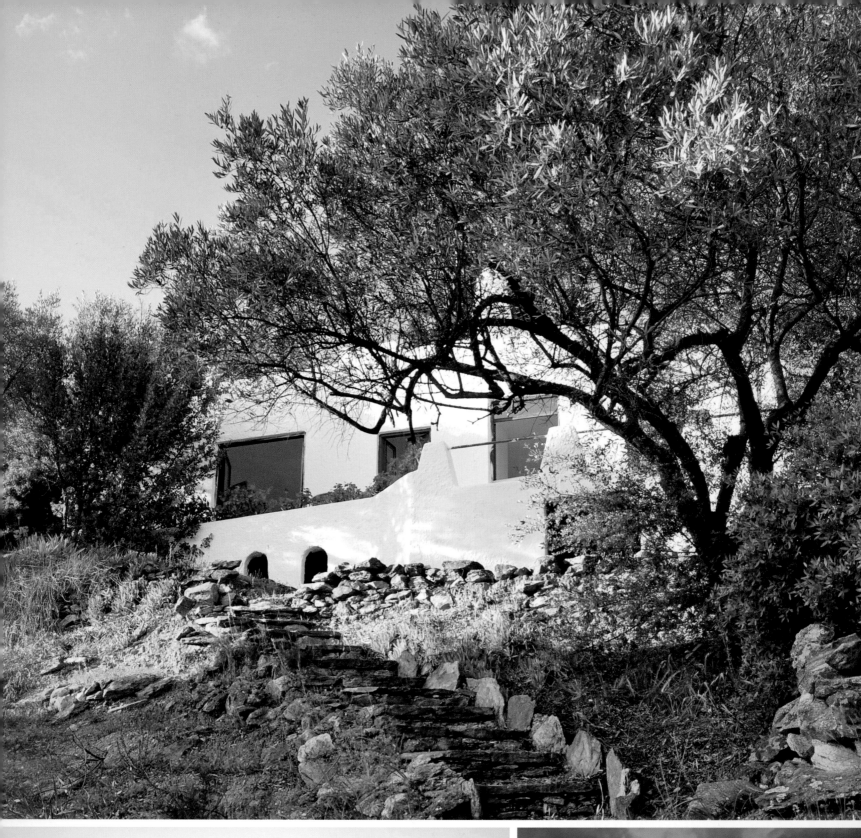

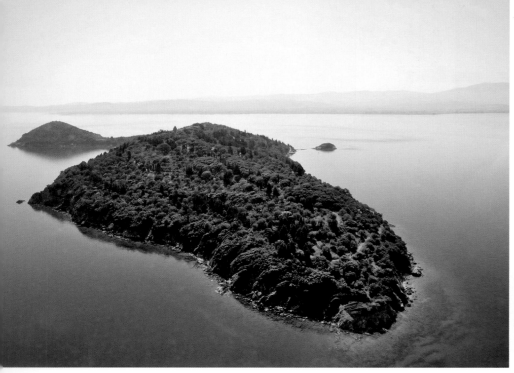

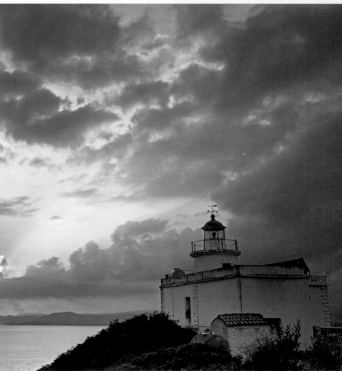

from above to below, from left to right: villa, aerial view,
lighthouse at sunrise

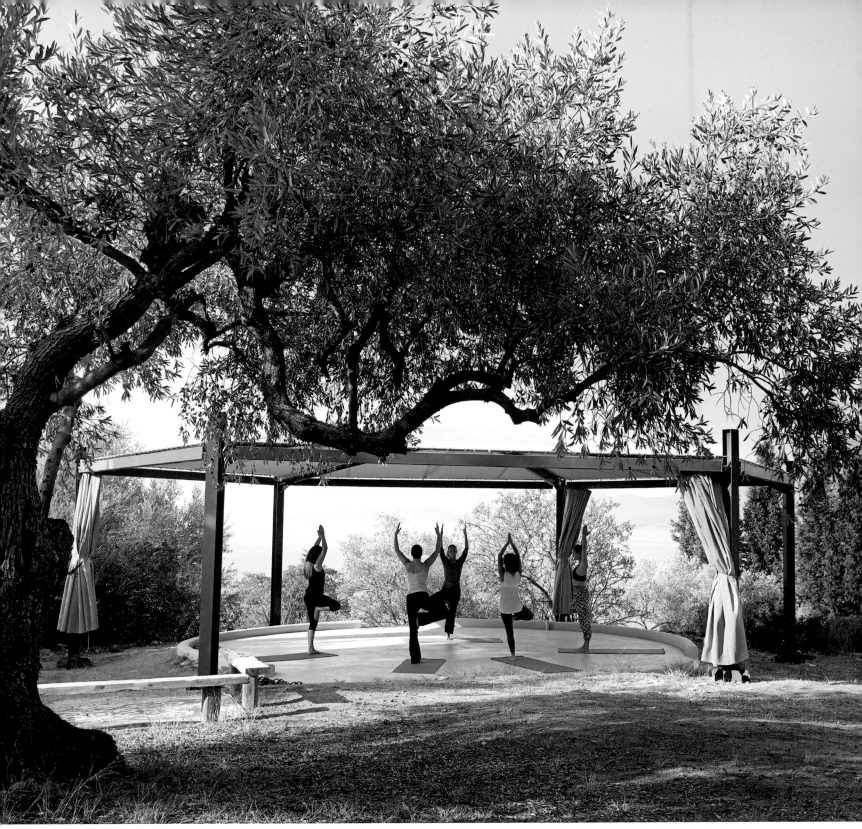

Yoga Shala tree & pavilion

Silver Island Yoga

Gulf of Volos, Greece

Designer: Claire and Lissa Christie
Location: private island, Gulf of Volos, Aegean sea, Greece
Year of completion: 2012
Area: 242,800 sqm
Type of retreat: spiritual, Buddhist meditation retreat

Silver Island is a privately owned, untouched dream island offering amost unique yoga experience. Situated a few miles from the mainland, Silver Island has been the Christie family home for fifty years. It has now opened its doors and sublime tranquility to those in search of a sense of inner peace and an escape from the hustle and bustle of modern life. The facility is a small and exclusive retreat accommodating up to ten guests in five beautifully decorated and inviting rooms. During the day the pebbled beaches, hidden coves and miles of pathways offer a chance for guests to spend time alone in quiet reflection between the two hour dawn and sunset yoga classes.

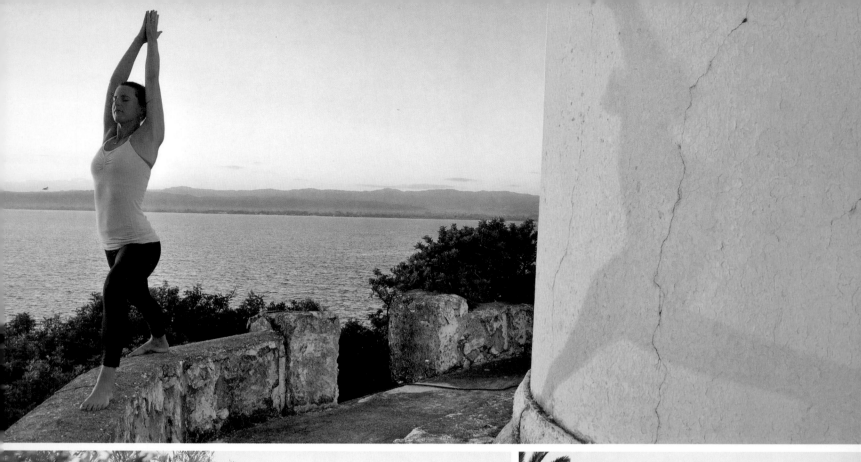

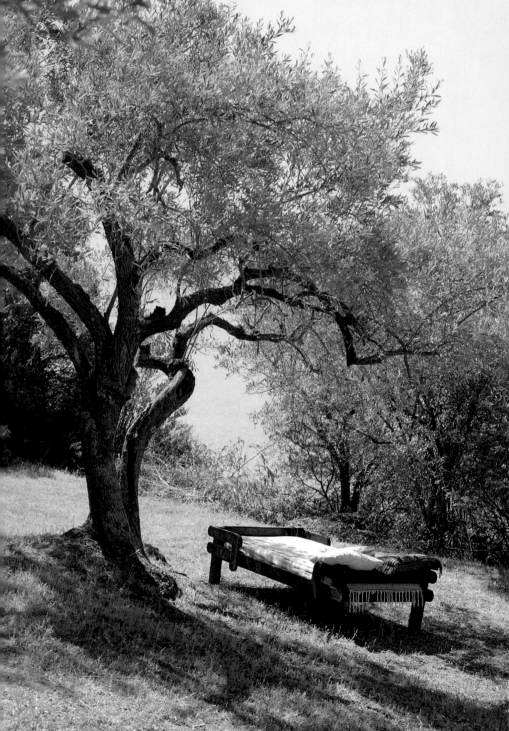

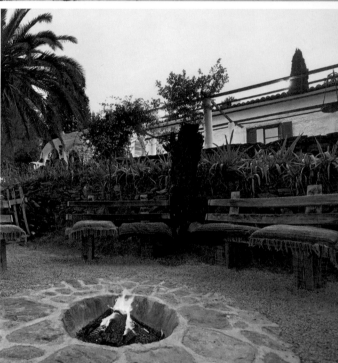

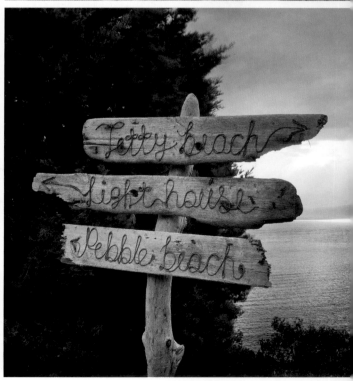

from above to below, from left to right: woman practicing yoga, daybed under tree, firepit, Silver Island signs

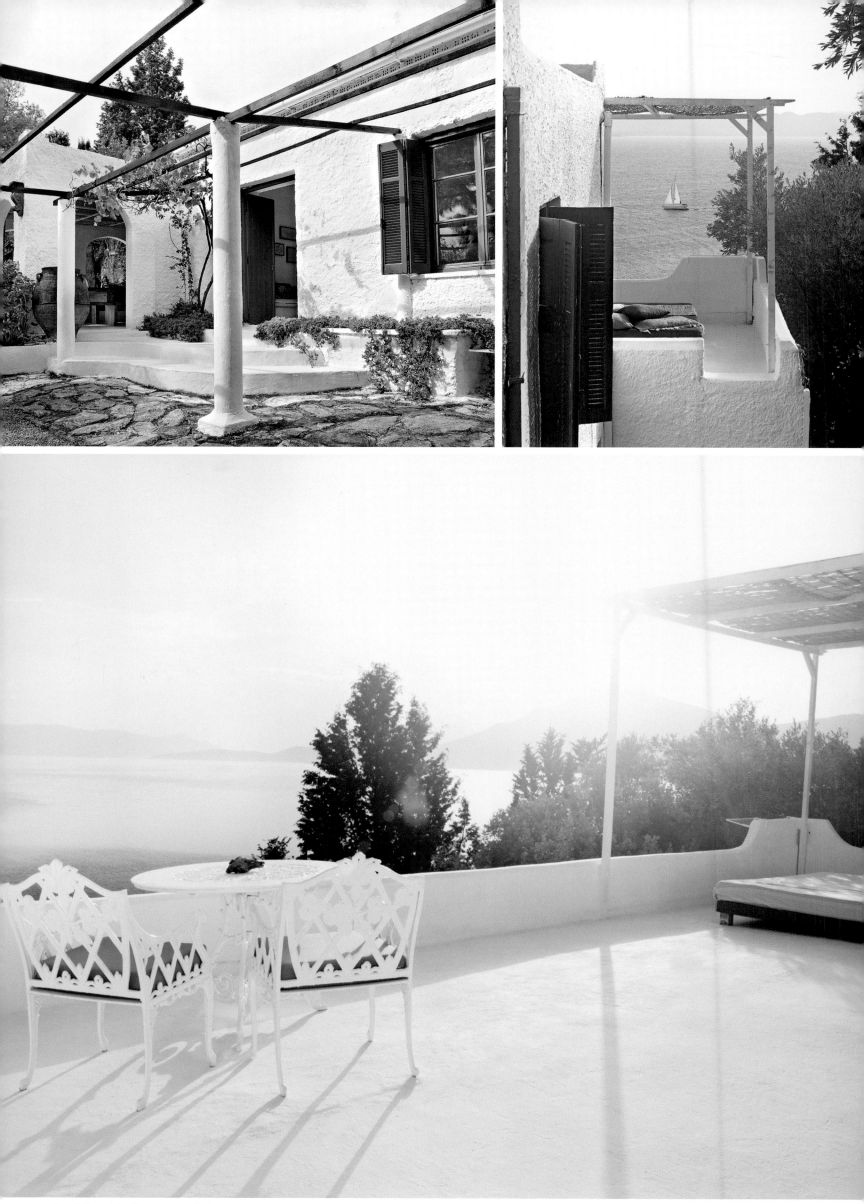

from left to right, from above to below: main house exterior,
boat view, balcony

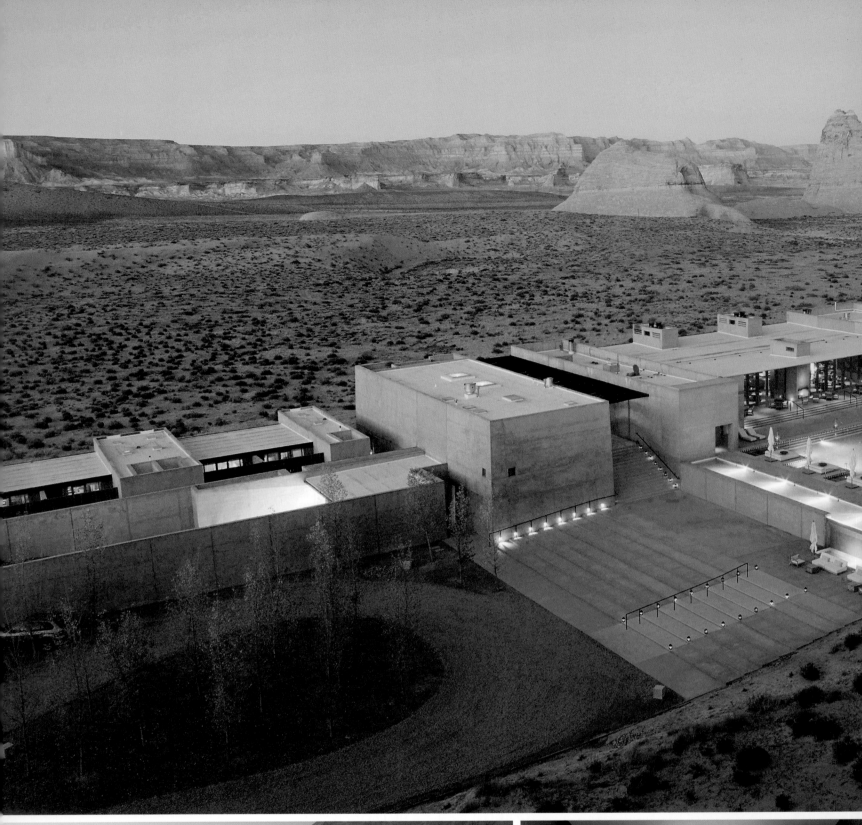

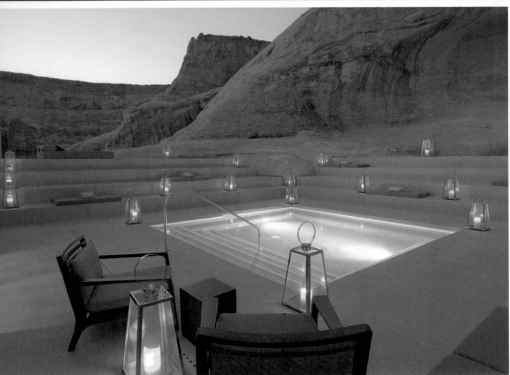

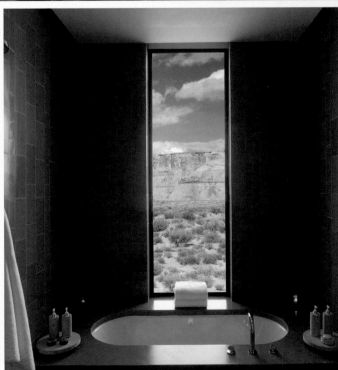

from above to below, from left to right: aerial view, spa step pool, suite bathroom

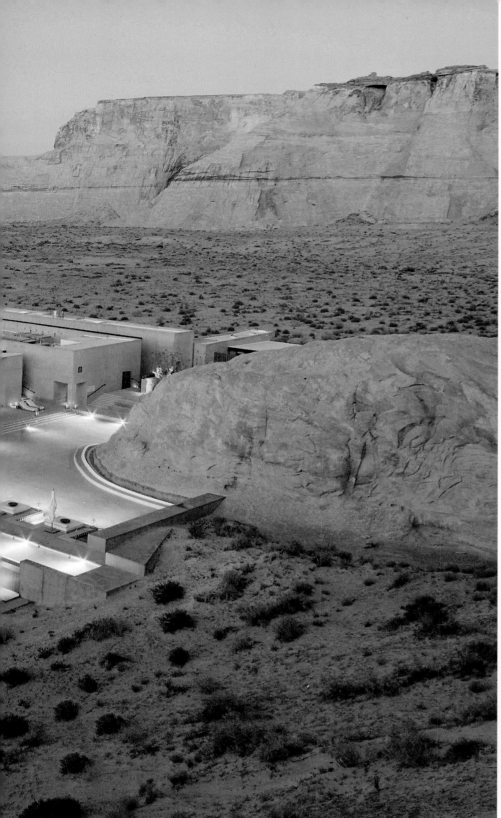

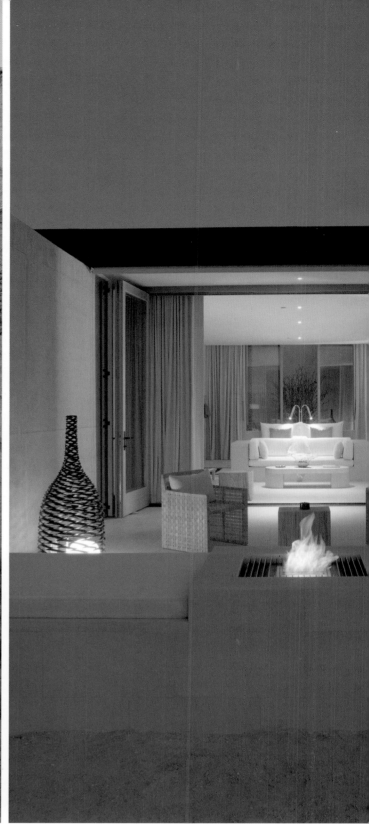

Girijaala suite

Amangiri

Utah, USA

Architect:
· Marwan Al-Sayed,
Wendell Burnette &
Rick Joy – I 10 studio
Location: 1 Kayenta Road,
Canyon Point,
Utah, USA
Year of completion: 2009
Type of retreat: resort

Amangiri is tucked into a protected valley with views over colorful, stratified rocks. Architecturally, the resort has been designed to blend into the landscape with natural hues, materials and textures. Although the structures are commanding and in proportion with the scale of the natural surroundings, they provide an intimate setting from which to view the landscape. Built around the main

swimming pool, the central pavilion embraces a dramatic stone escarpment. Within the pavilion are the living room, gallery, library, dining room, private dining room and cellar. Two accommodation wings lead from the pavilion into the desert: the Desert Wing with sixteen suites and the Mesa Wing with eighteen suites and Aman Spa.

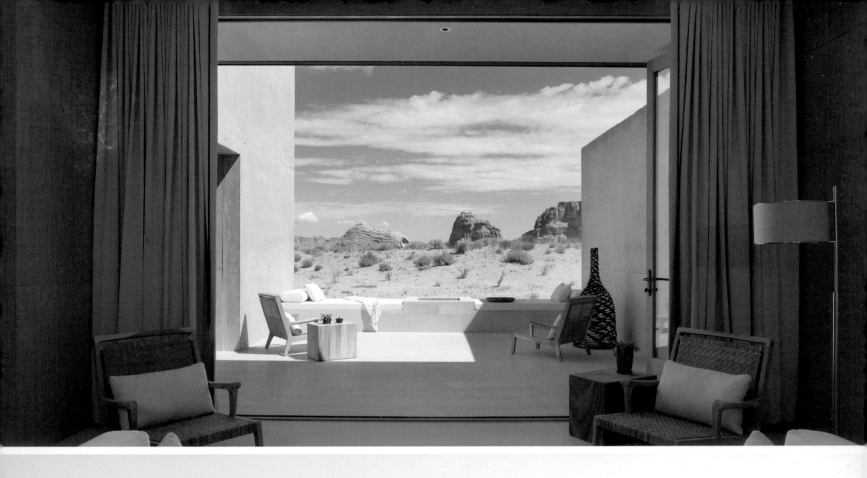

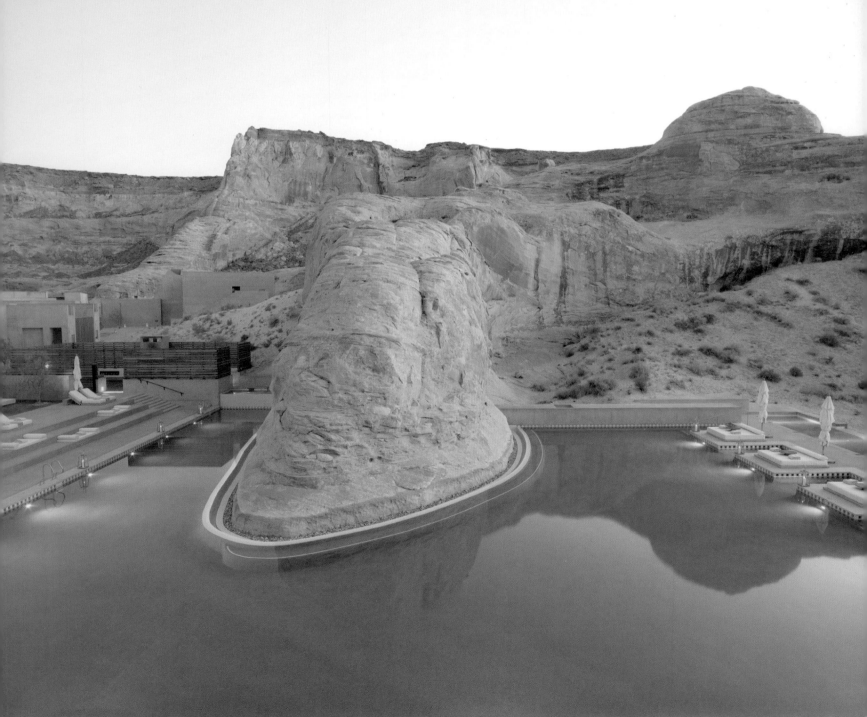

from above to below: terrace view, swimming pool

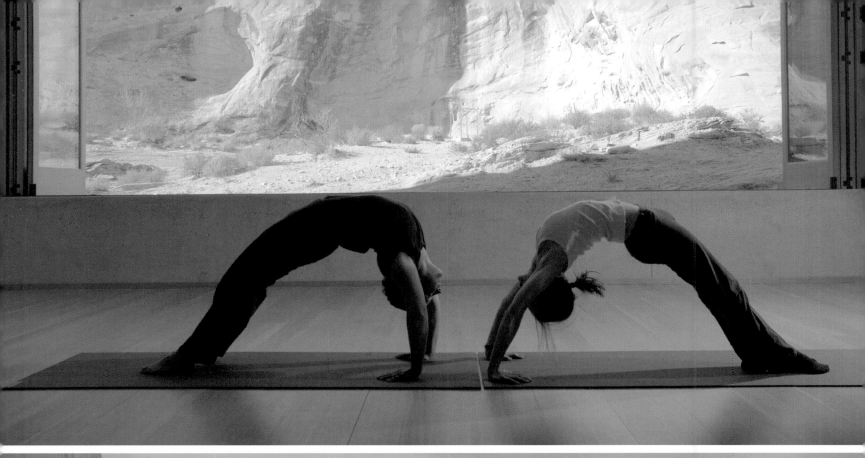

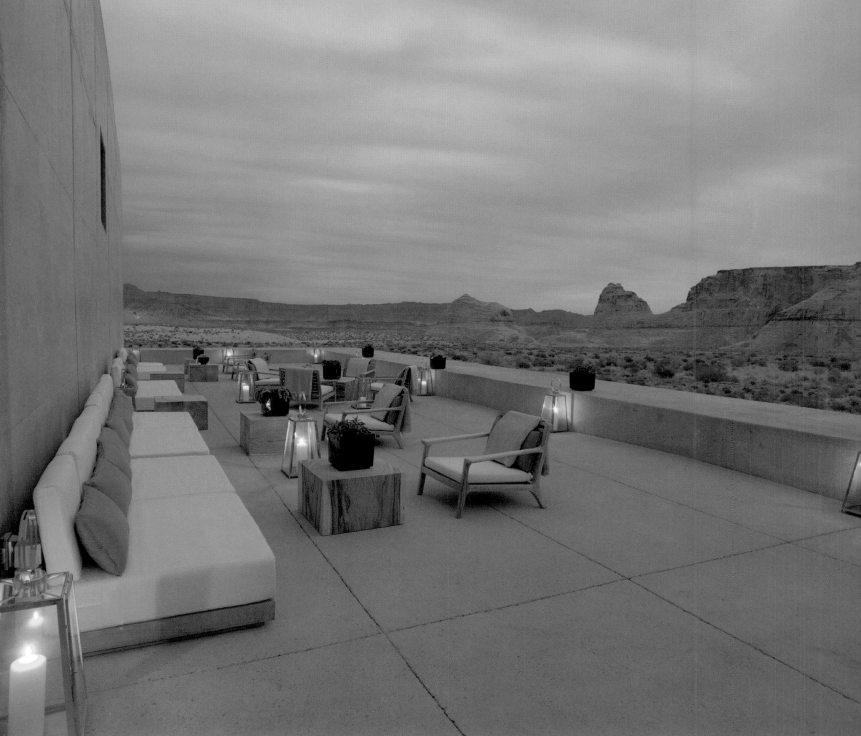

from above to below: yoga pavilion, desert lounge

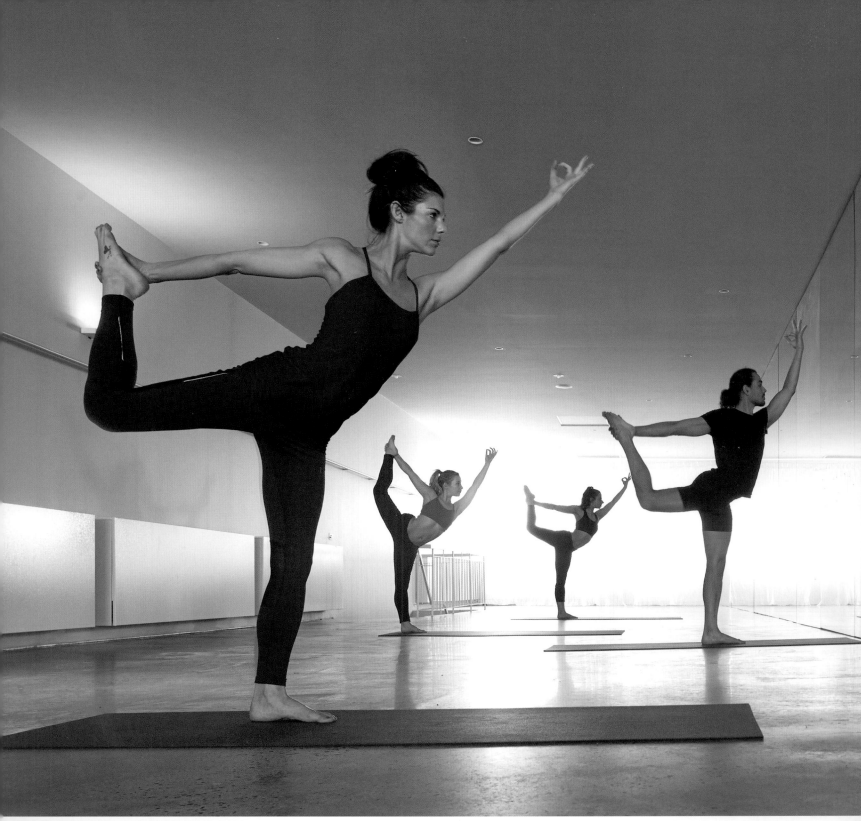

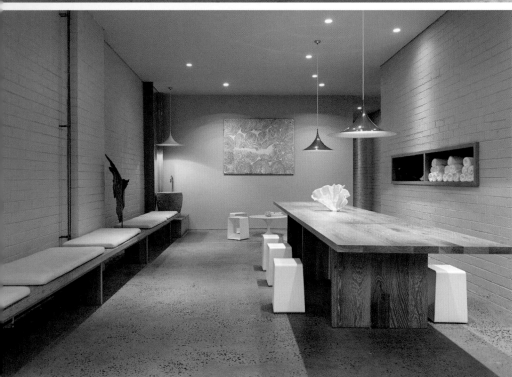

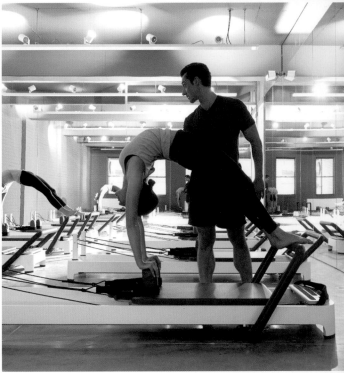

from above to below, from left to right: yoga space, reception, studio space

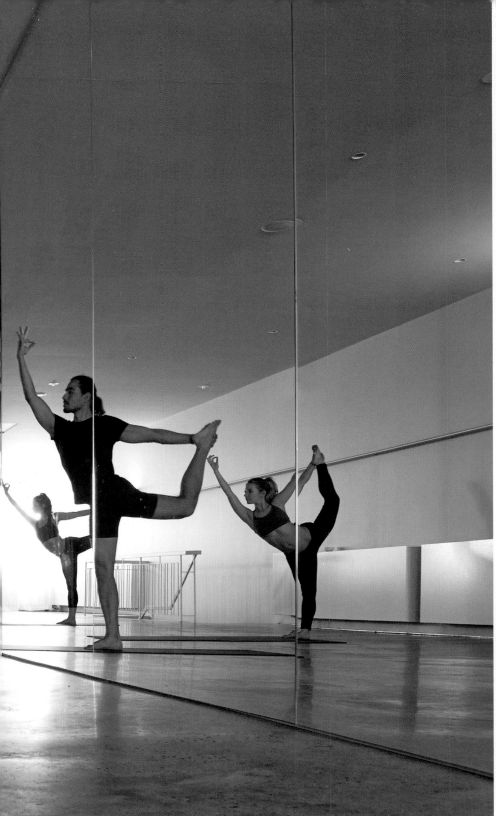
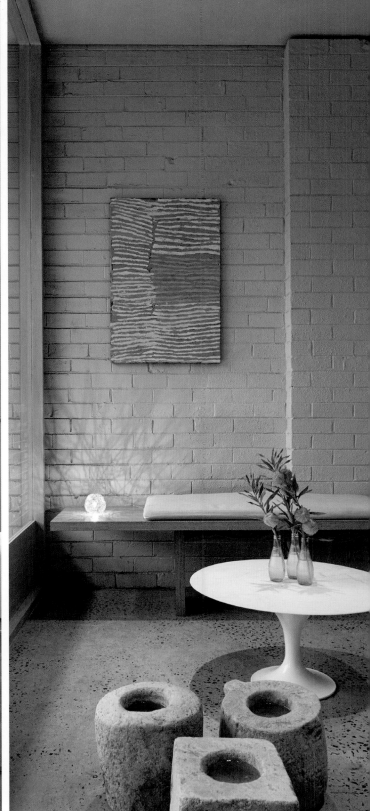

reception

One Hot Yoga & Pilates

Melbourne, Australia

Architect:
Robert Mills Architects and
Interior Designers
Location: South Yarra,
Melbourne, Australia
Year of completion: 2014
Area: 480 sqm
Type of retreat: yoga and
Pilates studio

The product of the marriage of an architect and a yogi, Rob and Lucinda Mills, One Hot Yoga & Pilates is a contemporary studio, an urban oasis in South Yarra, Melbourne. Founded in 2012, it was the first core body temperature Slow Hot Flow yoga studio in the world. In 2014 it has expanded the offering to include Power Flow Yoga, Yin Yoga, group Reformer Pilates and Hot Mat Pi-

lates classes. In addition it was introduced three additional studio spaces, hand-crafted and designed by Robert Mills Architects and Interior Designers. The One Hot Yoga & Pilates experience is based on the idea that at the point of connection between architecture, yoga and Pilates, the space we inhabit directly influences our physical and psychological wellbeing.

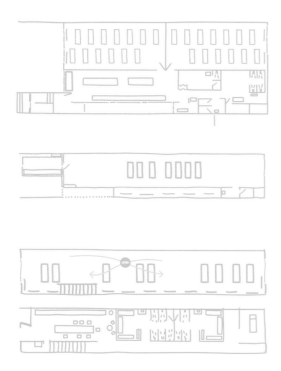

from above to below, from left to right: floor plans, changing room space, Pilates reception

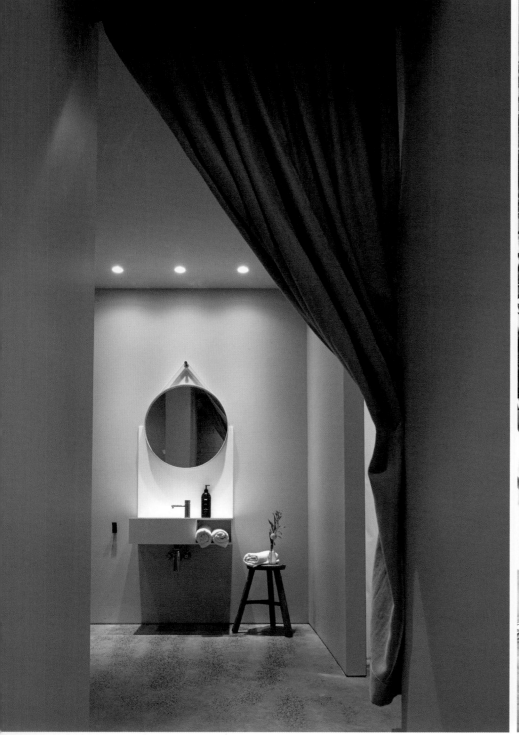

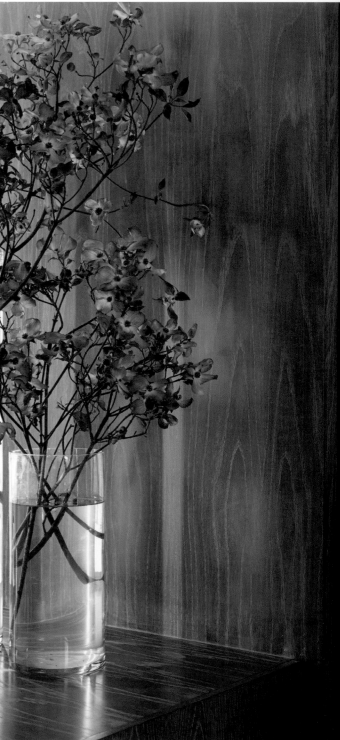

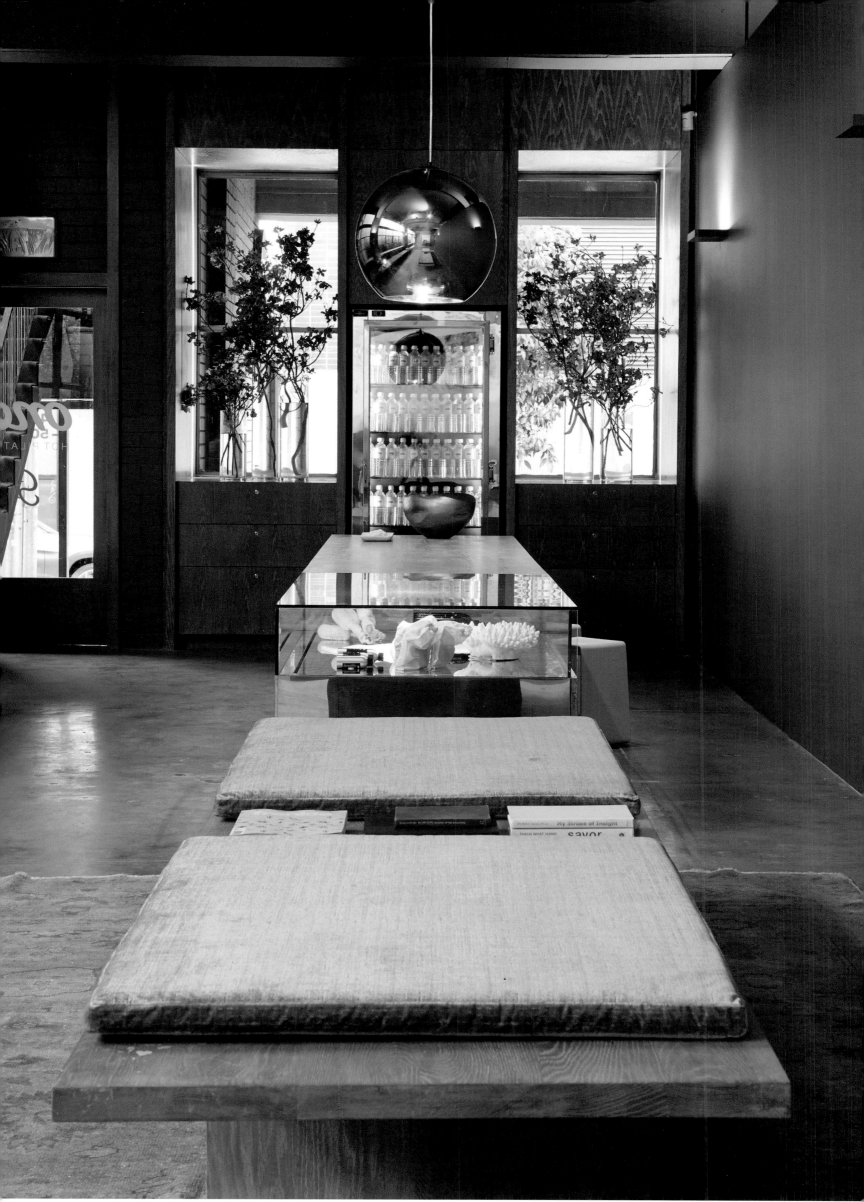

Pilates reception

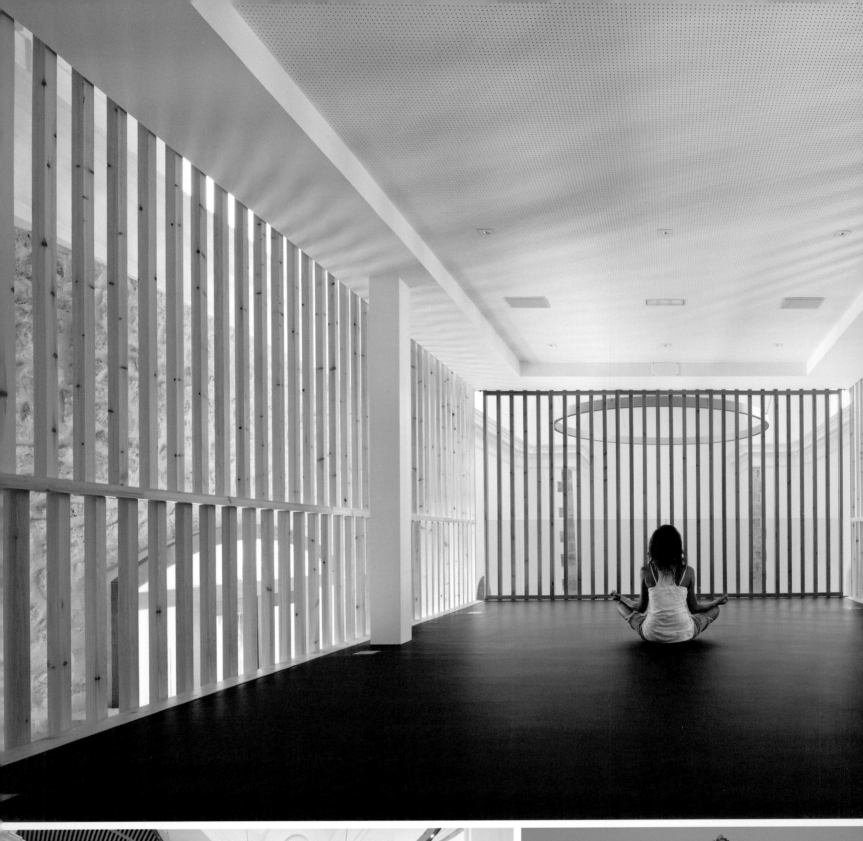

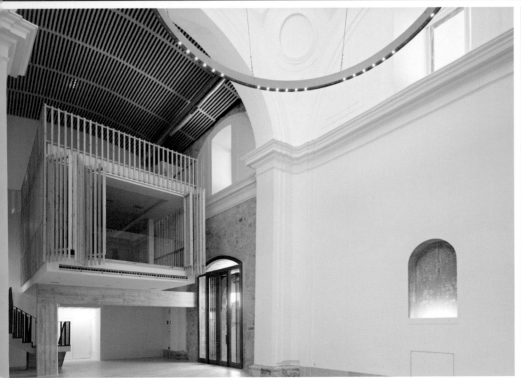

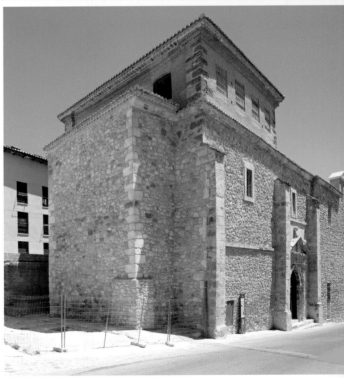

from above to below, from left to right: woman practicing yoga in
the choir loft, main space, exterior view

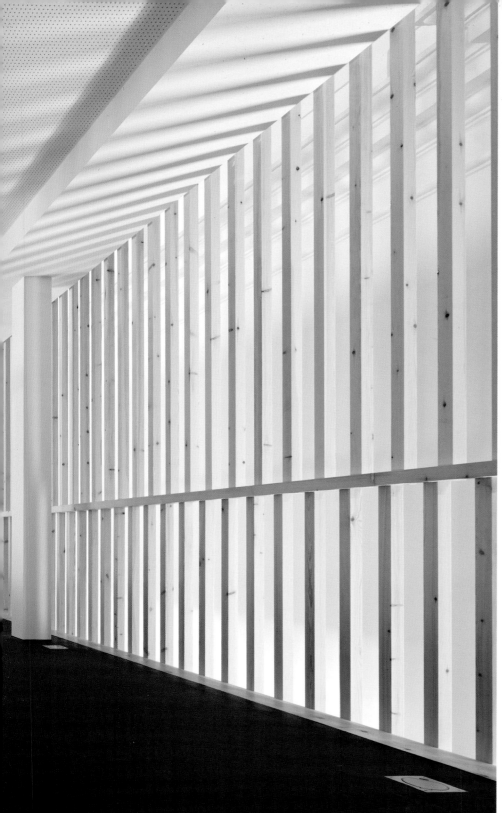
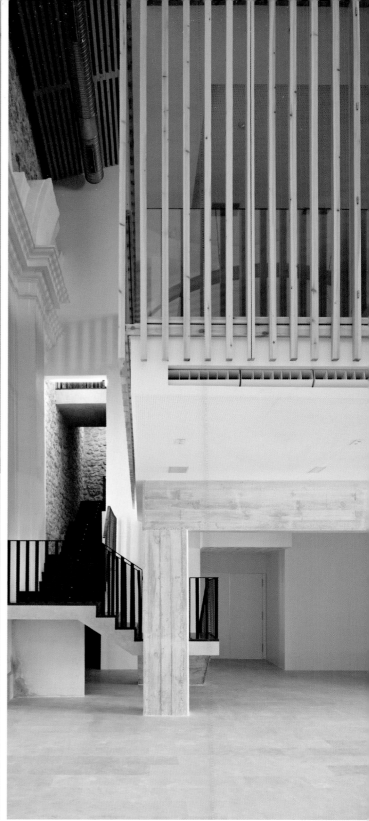

staircase

Chapel Rehabilitation

Brihuega, Spain

Architect:
Adam Bresnick architects
Location: Avenida
Constitución 4, 19400
Brihuega, Guadalajara, Spain
Year of completion: 2013
Area: 507 sqm
Type of retreat: religious

The chapel rehabilitation incorporates a multi-purpose space for events, ranging from a formal wedding to the mellow ambiance of a yoga retreat. The reconstruction involved healing complex pathologies suffered by the original structure after it was abandoned in 1969. Adam Bresnick architects studied and restored the existing architecture while inserting new uses. The philosophy guiding the intervention was to respect the passage of time. The stone façades were repointed, traditional tile eaves restored and stone moldings left with their worn faults. The original space has been restored, the entrance into the nave is a mix of archeological remains and new construction cantilevered over the space, minimally impinging on the original.

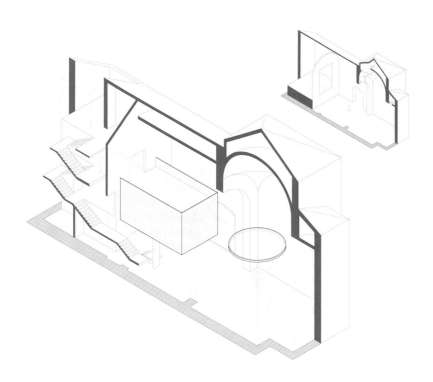

from above to below: isometric view, upper floor

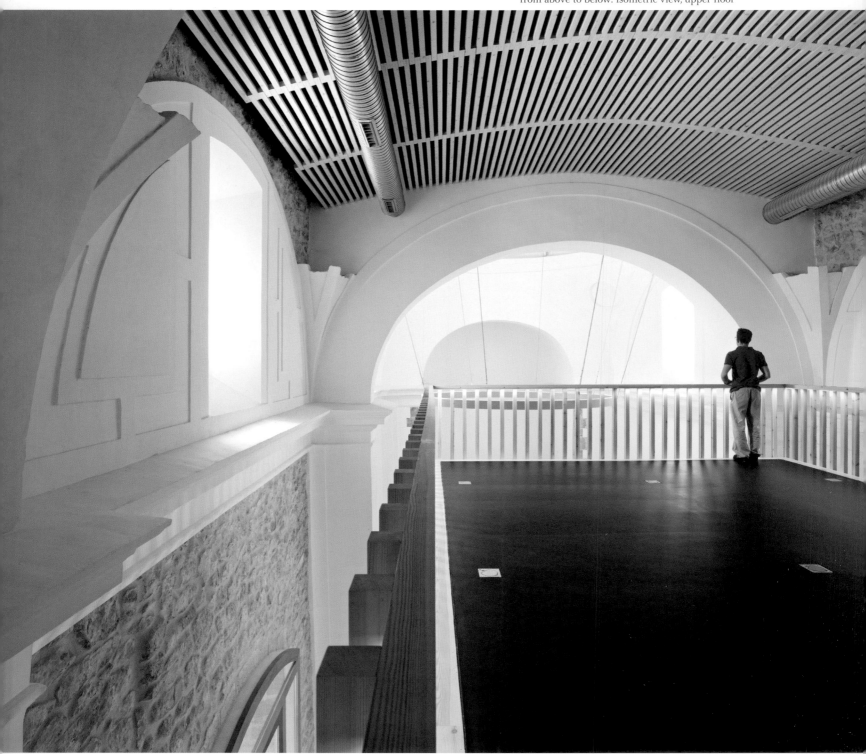

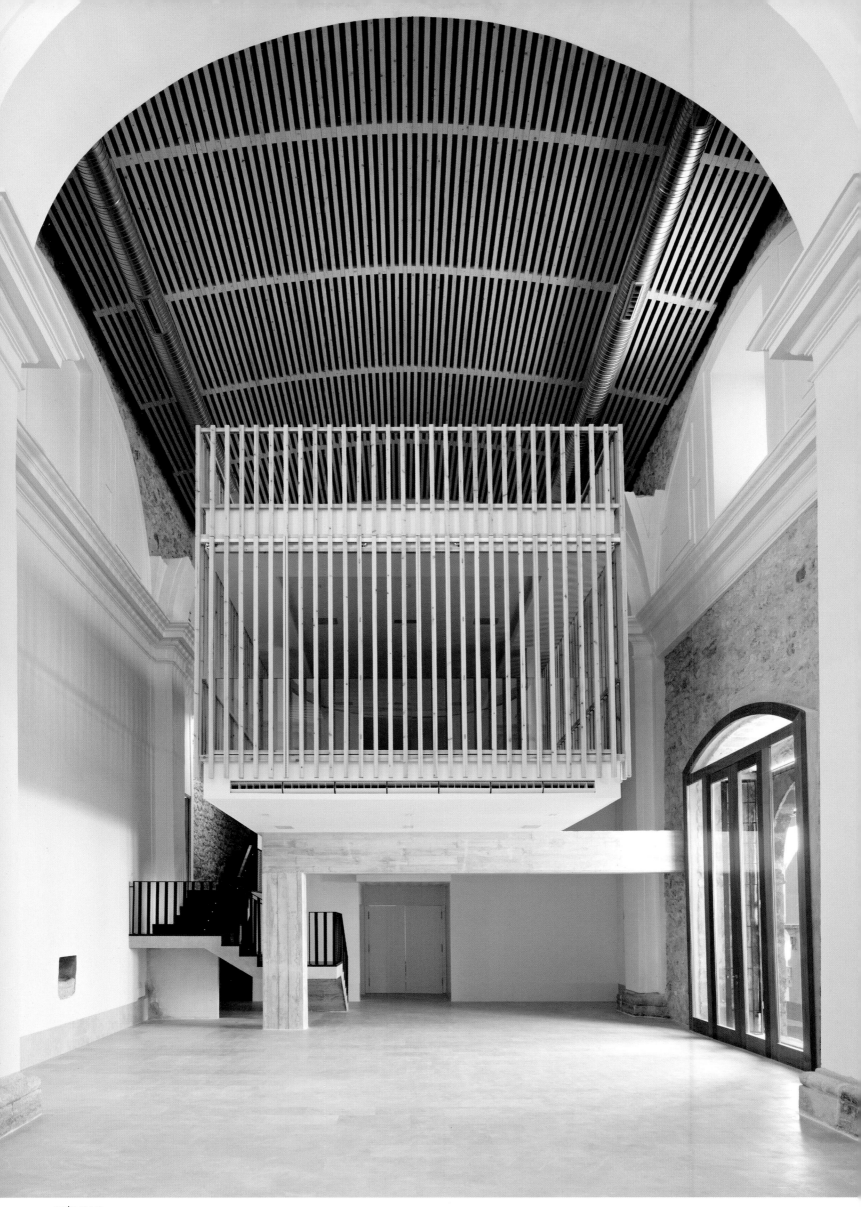

main space

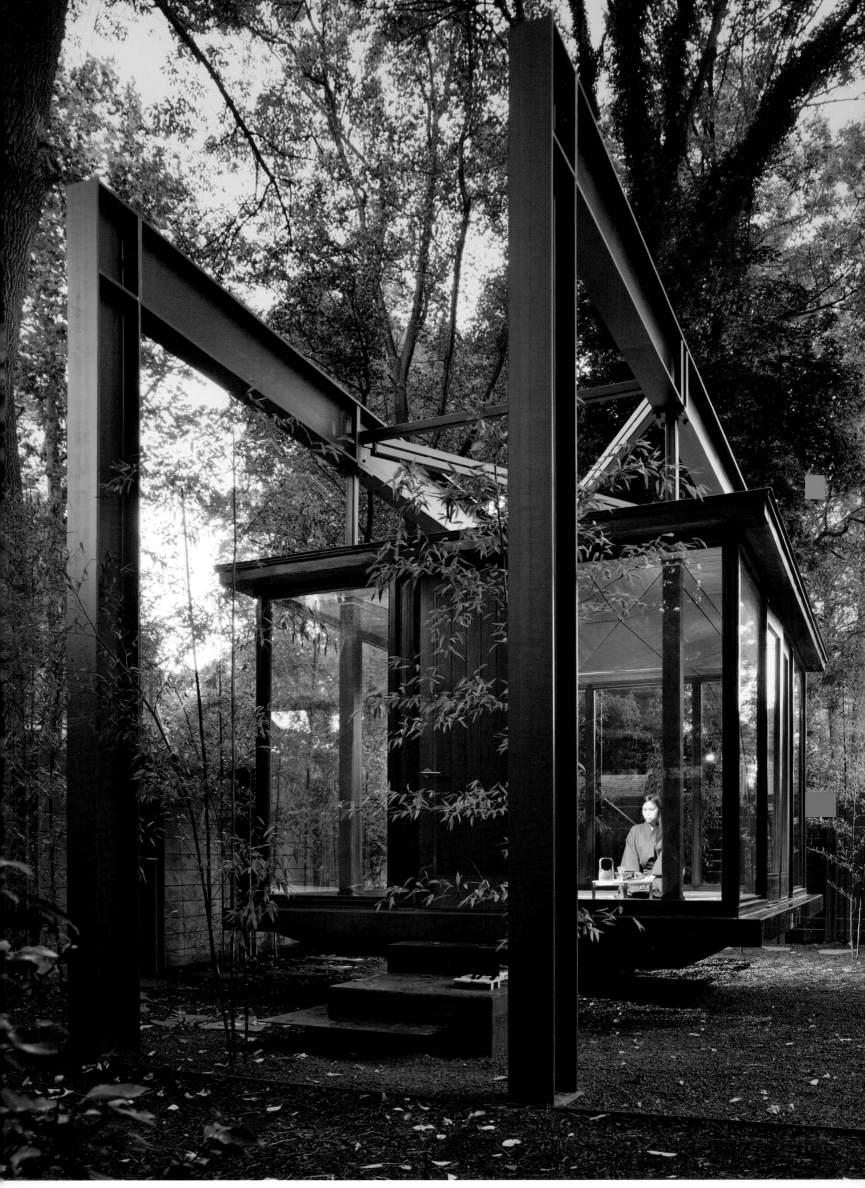

exterior view

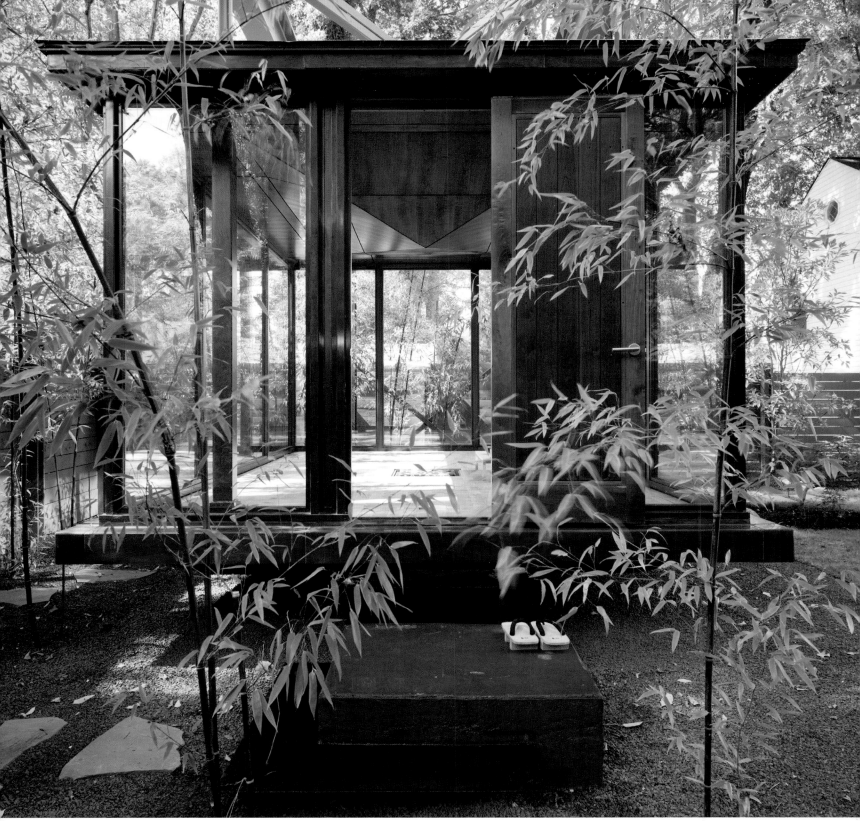

entrance

Tea House

Maryland, USA

Architect:
David Jameson Architect
Location: Bethesda,
Maryland, USA
Year of completion: 2009
Area: 14 sqm
Type of retreat:
meditation pavilion

A hanging bronze and glass object inhabits the backyard of a suburban home. The structure, which evokes the image of a Japanese lantern, acts as a tea house, meditation space, and stage for family musical recitals. Experiencing the image of the lantern as a singular gem floating in the landscape, funnels one into a curated procession space between strands of bamboo conceived to cleanse the mind in preparation to enter the object. After ascending an origami stair, the visitor is confronted with the last natural element: a four inch thick, opaque wood entry door. The visitor now occupies the structure as a performer with a sense of otherworldly meditation.

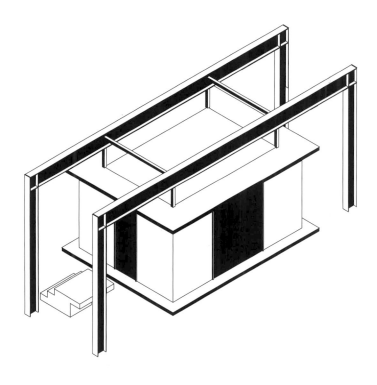

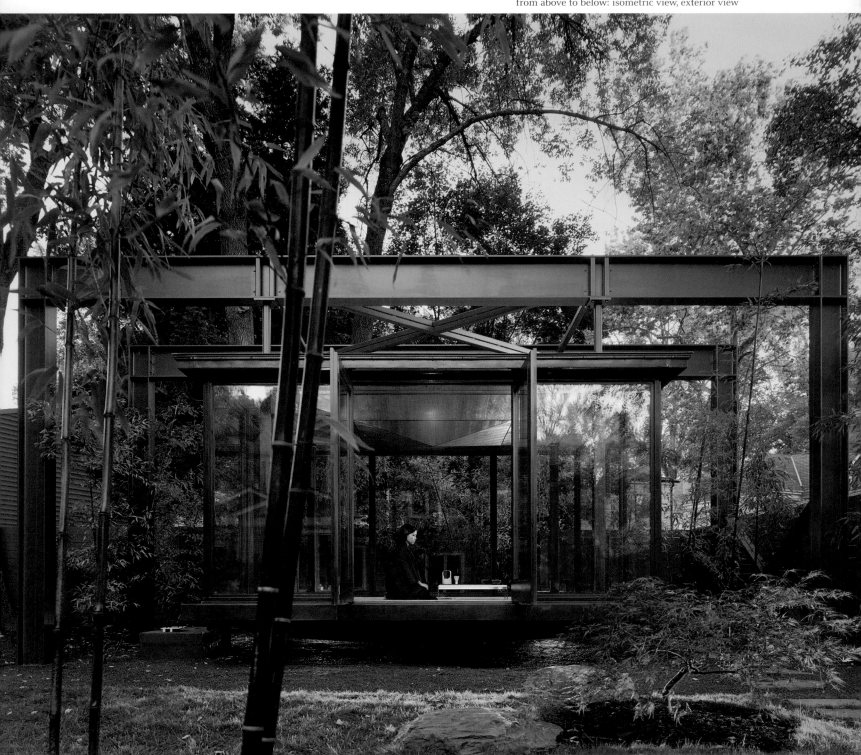

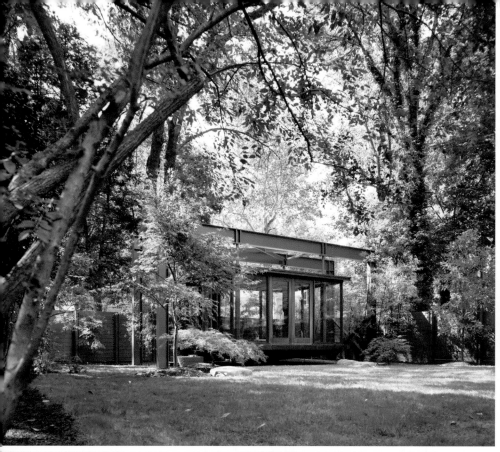

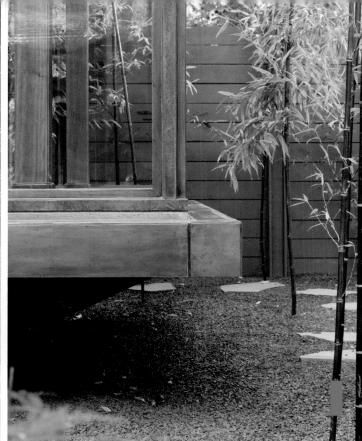

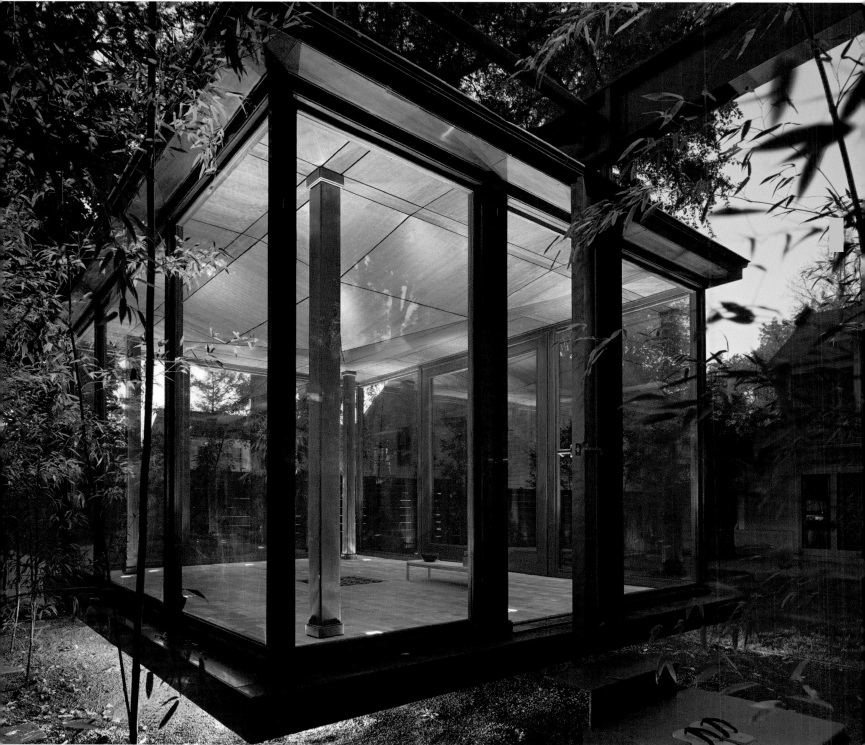

from left to right, from above to below: garden view, detail of
the façade, glass corner

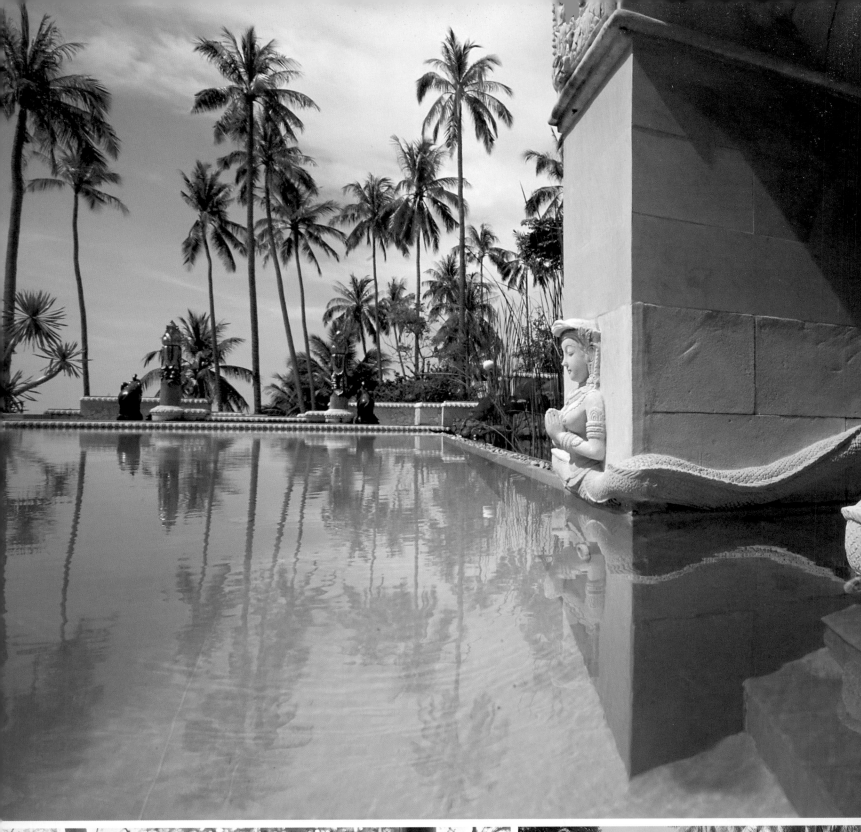

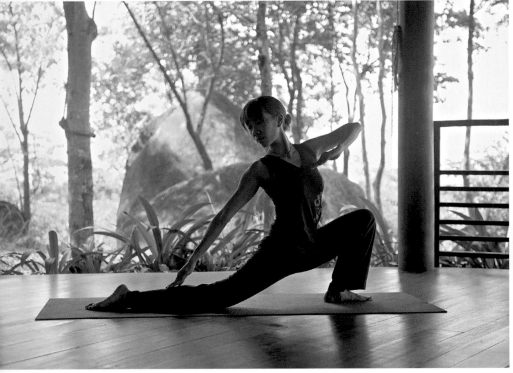

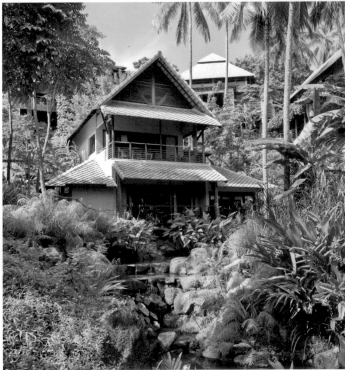

from above to below, from left to right: main pool, woman practicing yoga, ocean view villa

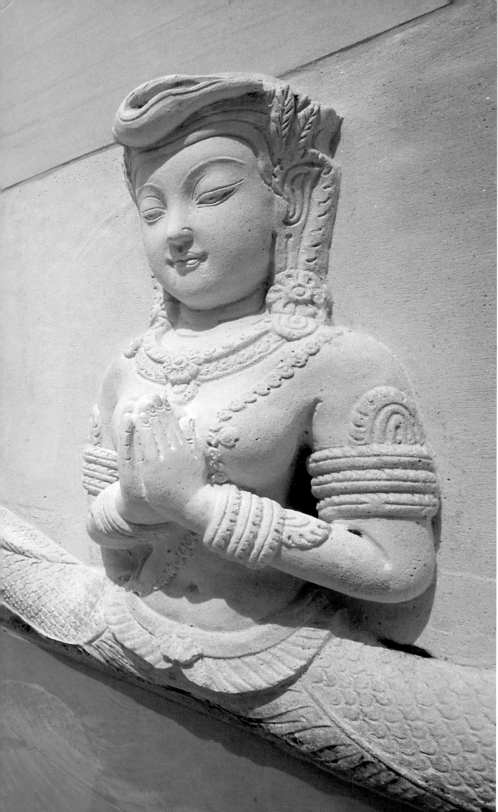

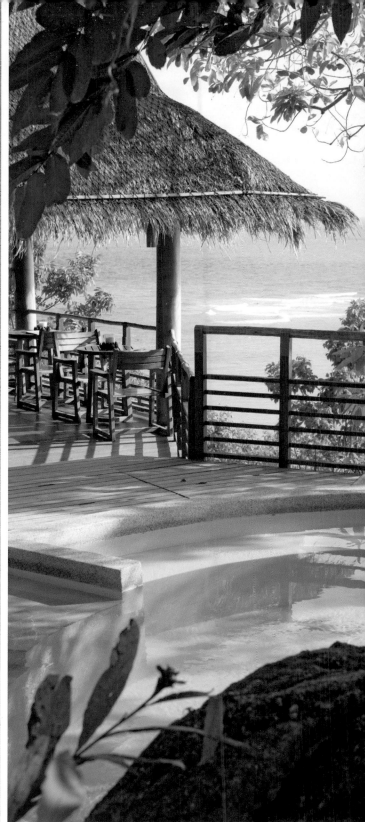

wellness elixir bar

Kamalaya Koh Samui

Koh Samui, Thailand

Architect:
Robert Powell
Location: Laem Set Beach,
Na-Muang, Koh Samui,
Suratthani 84140, Thailand
Year of completion: 2005
Area: 40,000 sqm
Type of retreat:
spiritual resort

Kamalaya is a multi-award winning Wellness Sanctuary and Holistic Spa located on the southern coast of Koh Samui, Thailand. Founded by John and Karina Stewart in 2005, the resort offers an holistic wellness experience that integrates healing therapies from East and West, a breathtakingly beautiful natural environment, inspired healthy cuisine and customized wellness programs rang-ing from Detoxification to Stress & Burnout, as well as Optimal Fitness, Sleep Enhancement, Yoga Synergy and Emotional Balance. Centered around a monk's cave that once served Buddhist monks as a place of spiritual re-treat, Kamalaya's name expresses its essence: "Lotus (ka-mal) Realm (alaya)", is an ancient symbol for the unfolding of the human spirit.

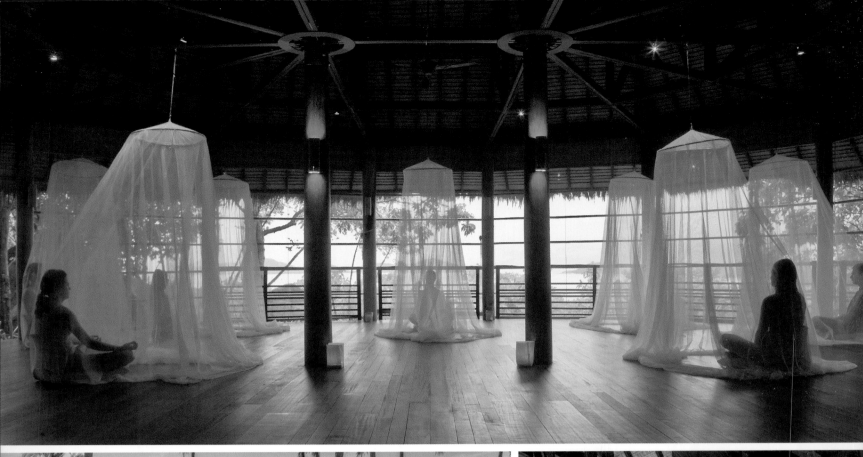

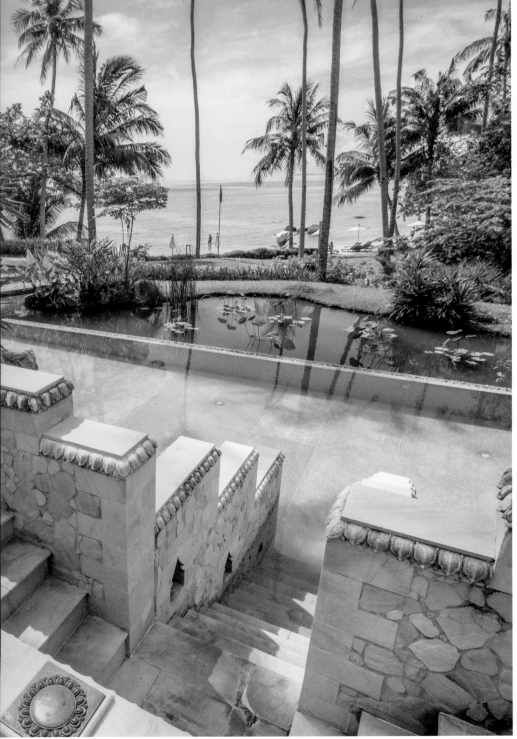

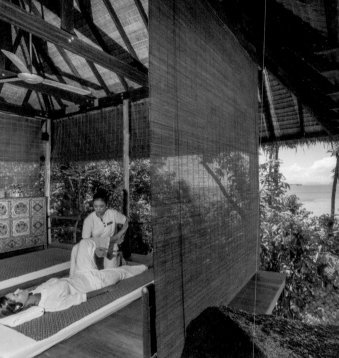

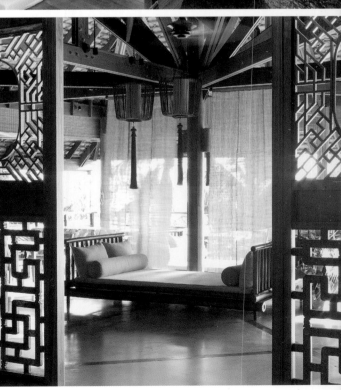

from above to below, from left to right: meditation pavilion,
Kamalaya leisure pool, open treatment room, Alchemy tea lounge

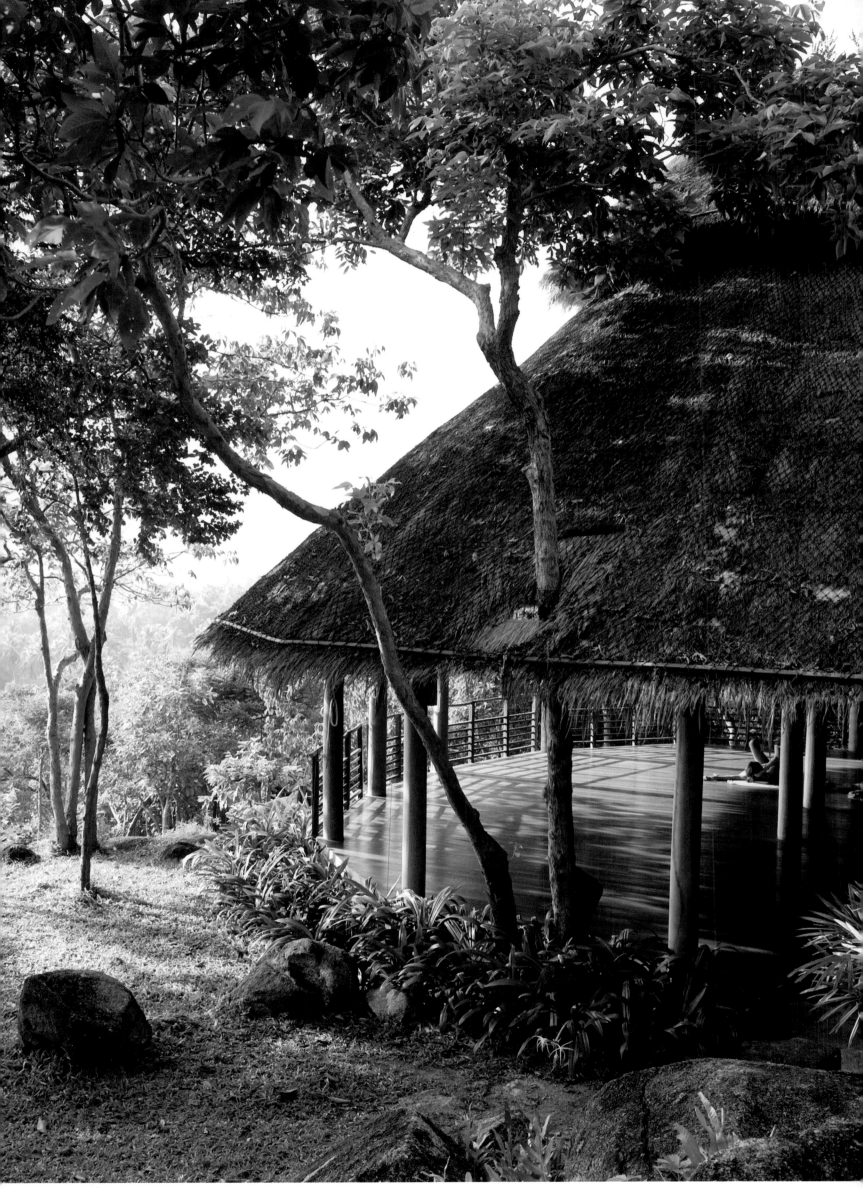

yoga pavilion

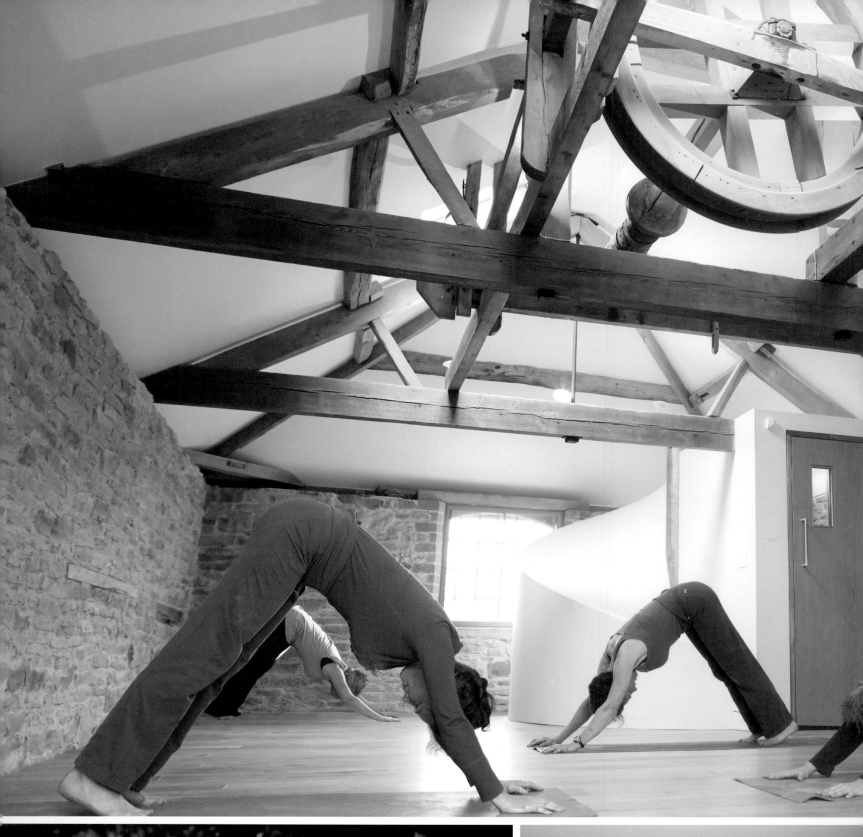

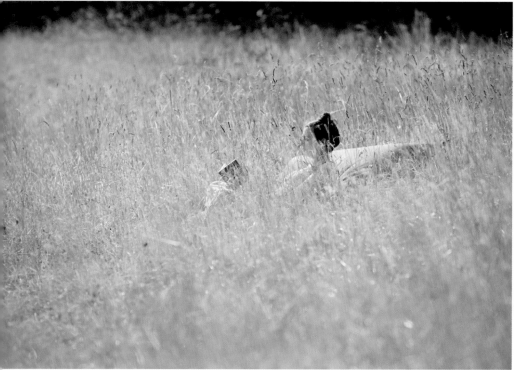

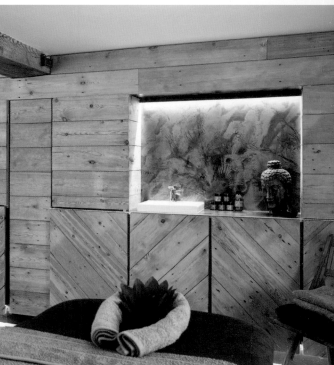

from above to below, from left to right: yoga studio in Mill Loft,
nothing to do, treatment room

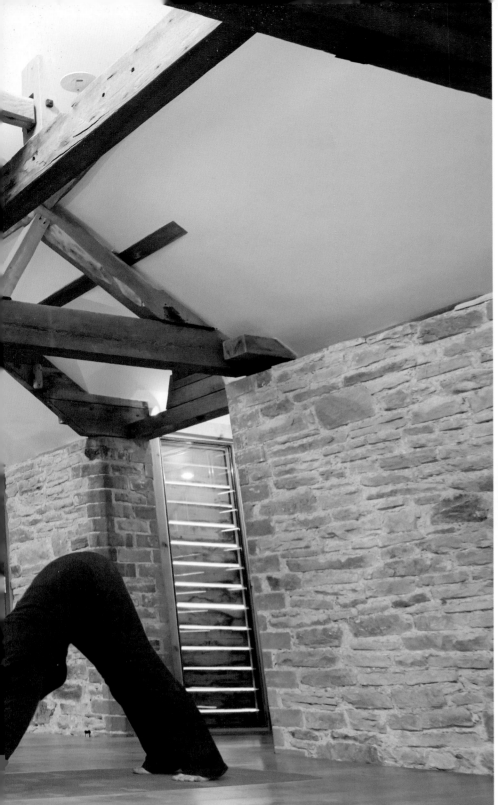
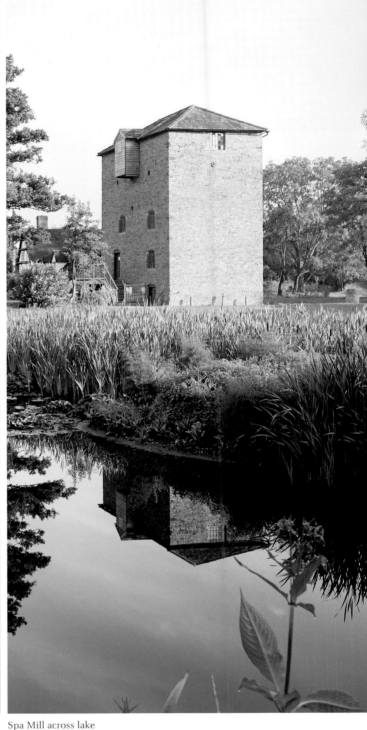

Spa Mill across lake

The Clover Mill

Herefordshire, United Kingdom

Architect: Craft Architects
Location: Cradley, Malvern, Worcestershire WR13 5NR, United Kingdom
Year of completion: 2013
Area: 475 sqm
Type of retreat: spa & yoga specializing in Ayurveda

The Clover Mill is the UK's first boutique Ayurvedic spa retreat, set in the natural untouched Herefordshire countryside with views of the Malvern Hills. At The Clover Mill you will find a beautiful restful retreat, with lavish and innovative eco-accommodation in lodges designed around ayurvedic Vastu principles to five star standards. It offers beautiful modern spa facilities, placed in harmony with the original milling equipment, to provide individualized treatments, yoga classes, meditation and dining founded on the ancient art and science of Ayurveda. As an ultimate wellbeing escape you can unwind and indulge in a relaxing ayurvedic treatment, spend a day in the spa or take a full retreat to detox and rejuvenate, immersed in nature.

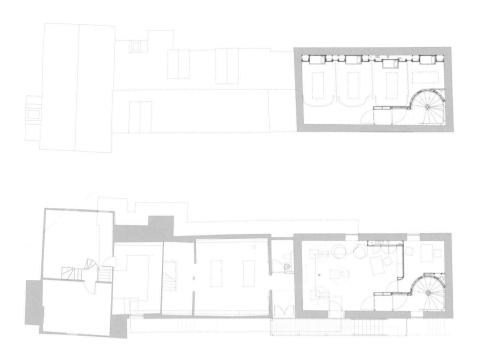

from above to below: floor plans, interior view

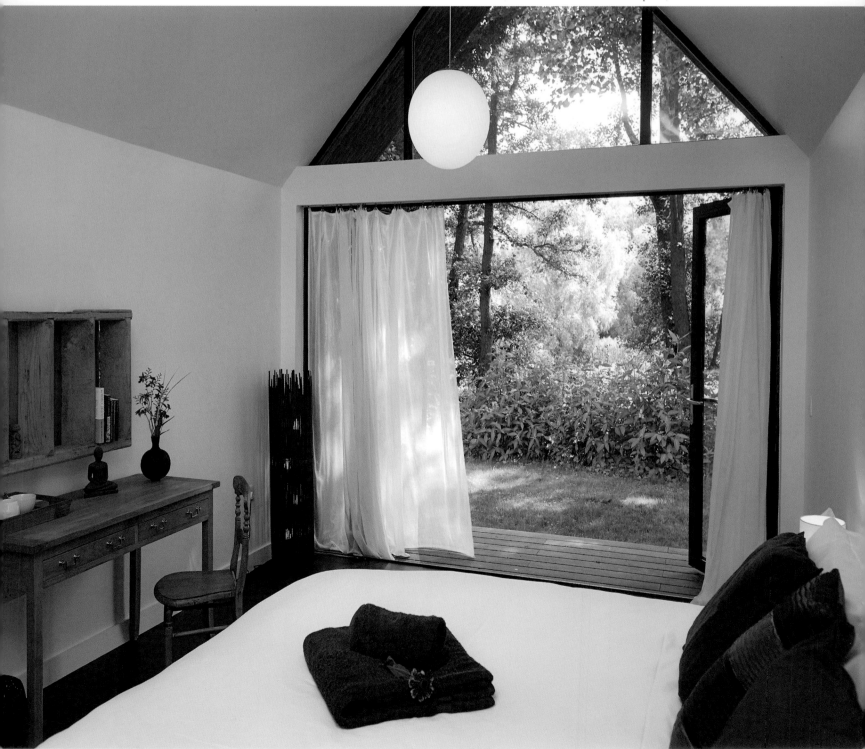

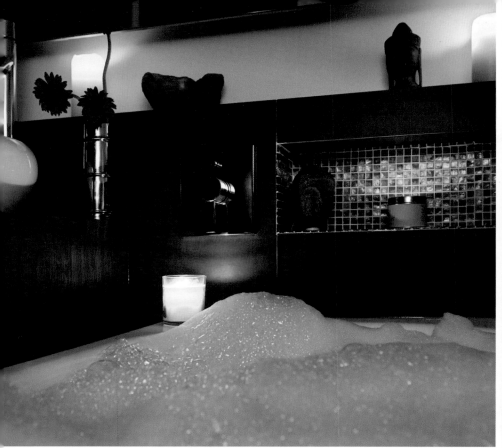

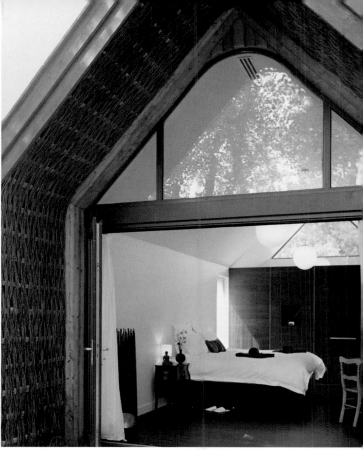

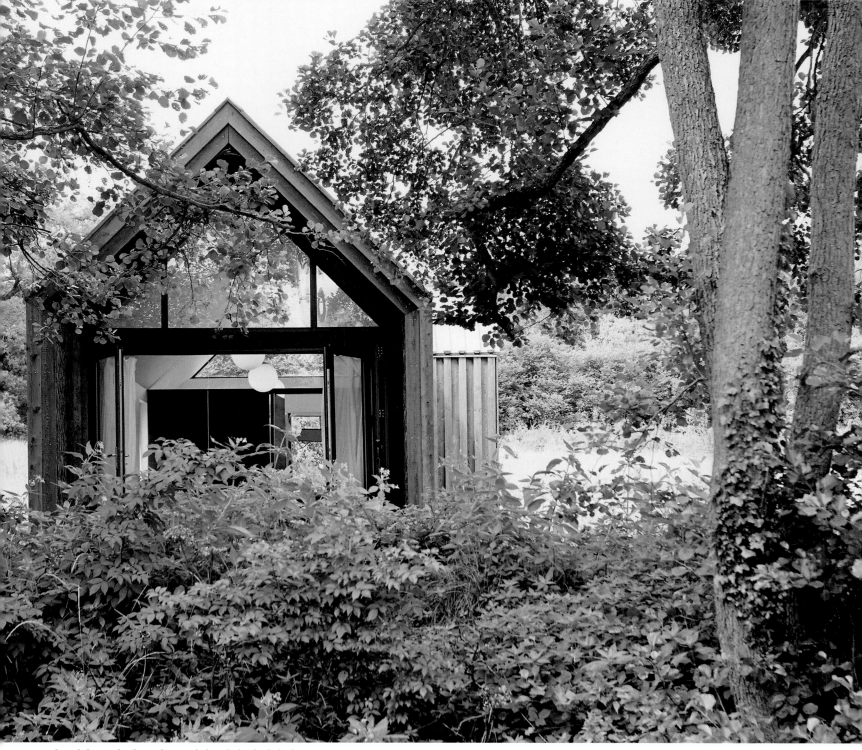

from left to right, from above to below: lodge bath, bedroom,
eco lodge

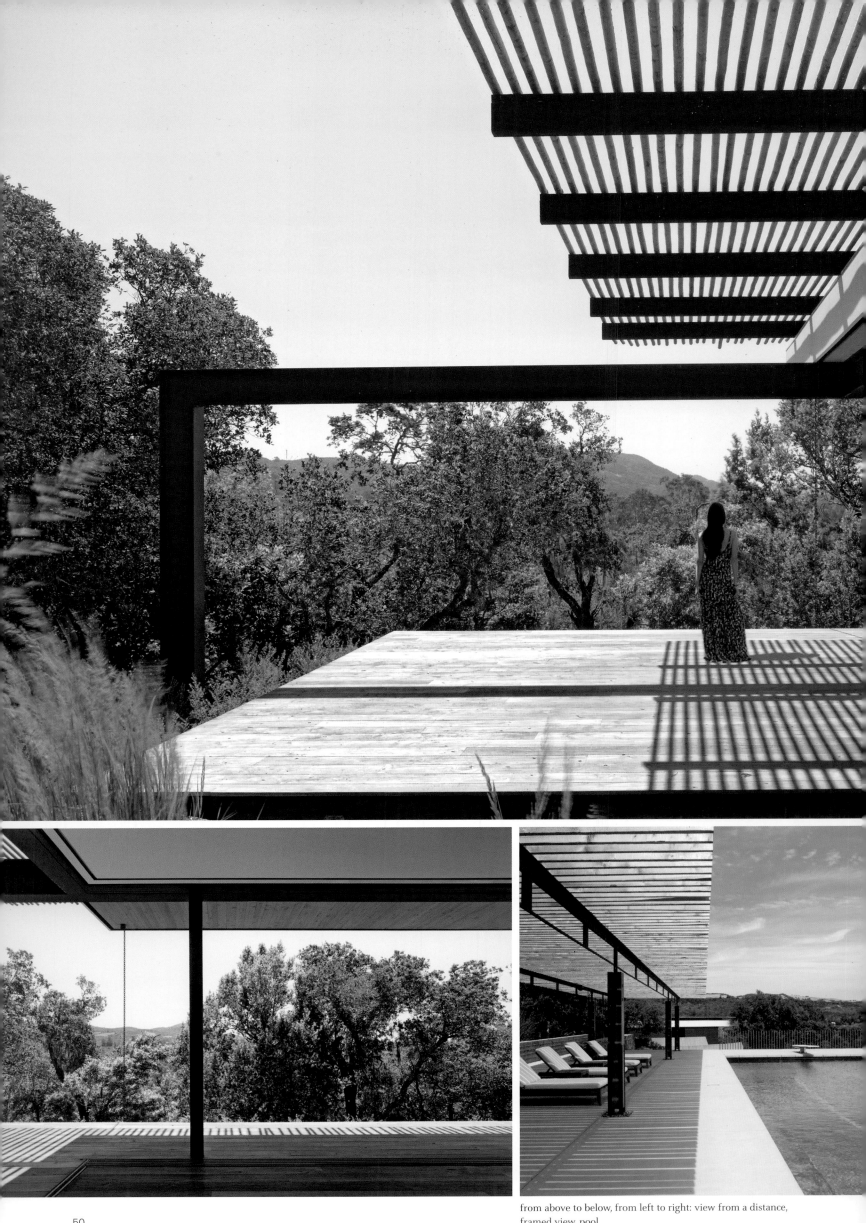

50

from above to below, from left to right: view from a distance, framed view, pool

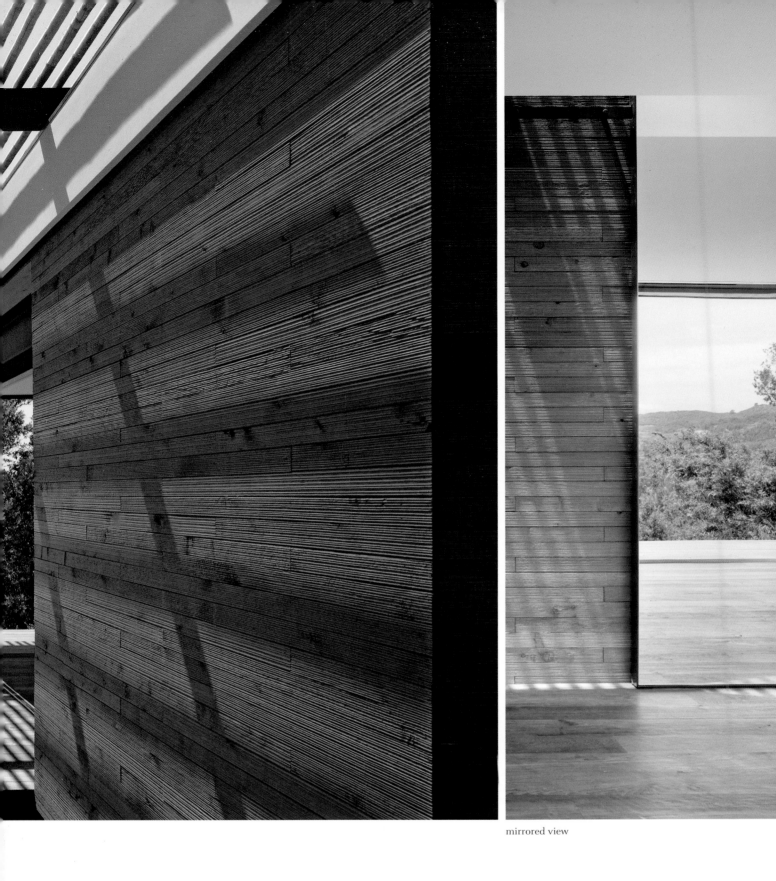
mirrored view

Sonoma Spa Retreat

Sonoma, USA

Architect:
Aidlin Darling Design
Location: Quarry Hill Road,
Sonoma, California, USA
Year of completion: 2009
Area: 102 sqm
Type of retreat: private
exercise, meditation
and relaxation space

Inherent in the idea of creating a retreat are concepts of privacy, safety and refuge. By creating a private space away from the frenetic rhythms of the everyday, the possibility emerges to relax, to reconnect with oneself and more completely understand the natural environment. It is through this separation from the everyday, this quieting of the mind, that a deeper connection with the self can

be achieved. The building seeks to foster self-discovery not only by creating a sense of privacy through its many protective layers, but once inhabited, aspires to retreat, leaving the inhabitant and nature to become reacquainted. The Sonoma Spa Retreat was created as a private exercise, meditation and relaxation space for a businessman and his family.

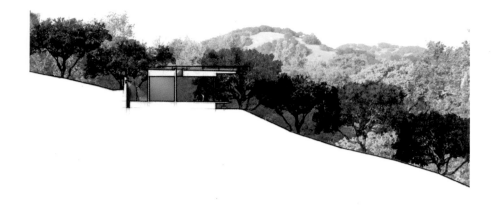

from above to below, from left to right: section, woman practicing yoga, dusk, ramp

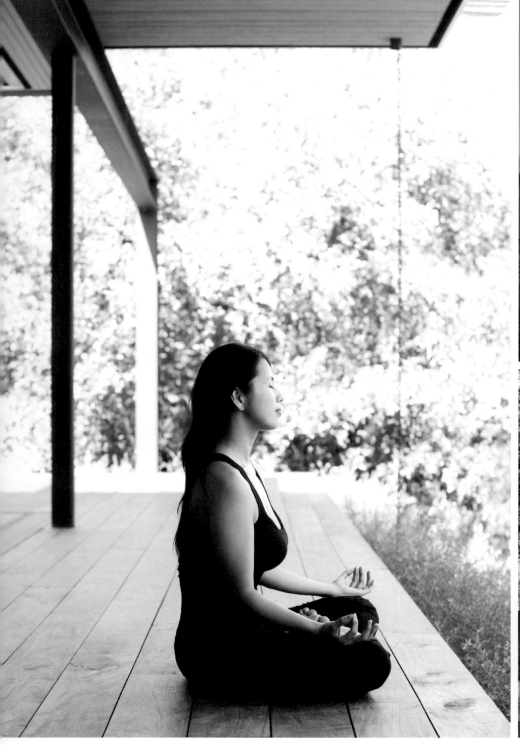

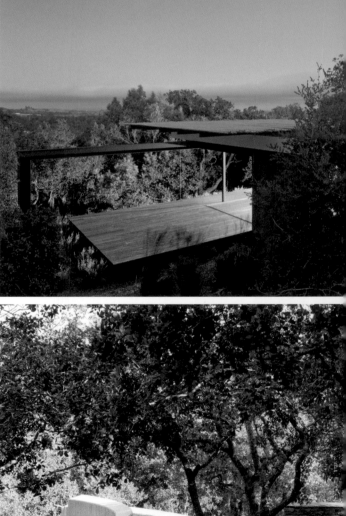

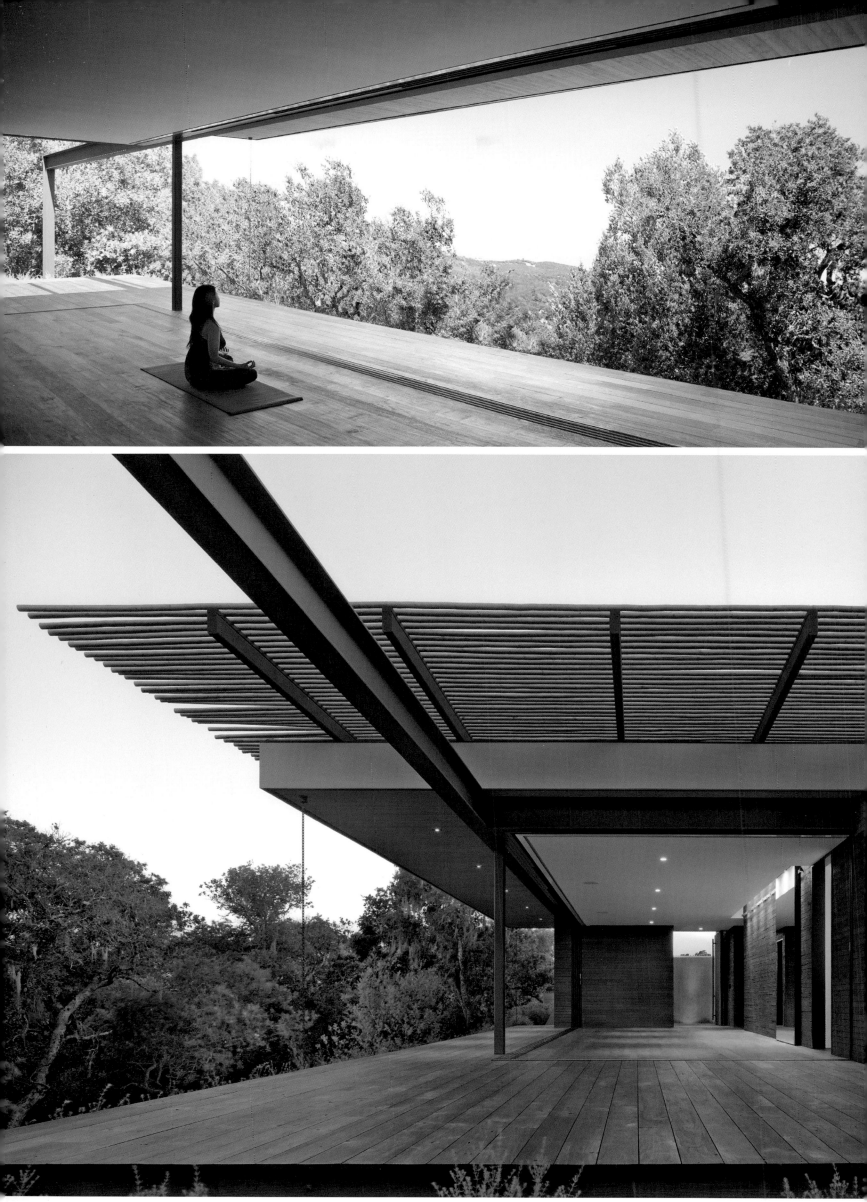

from above to below: woman practicing yoga, perspective

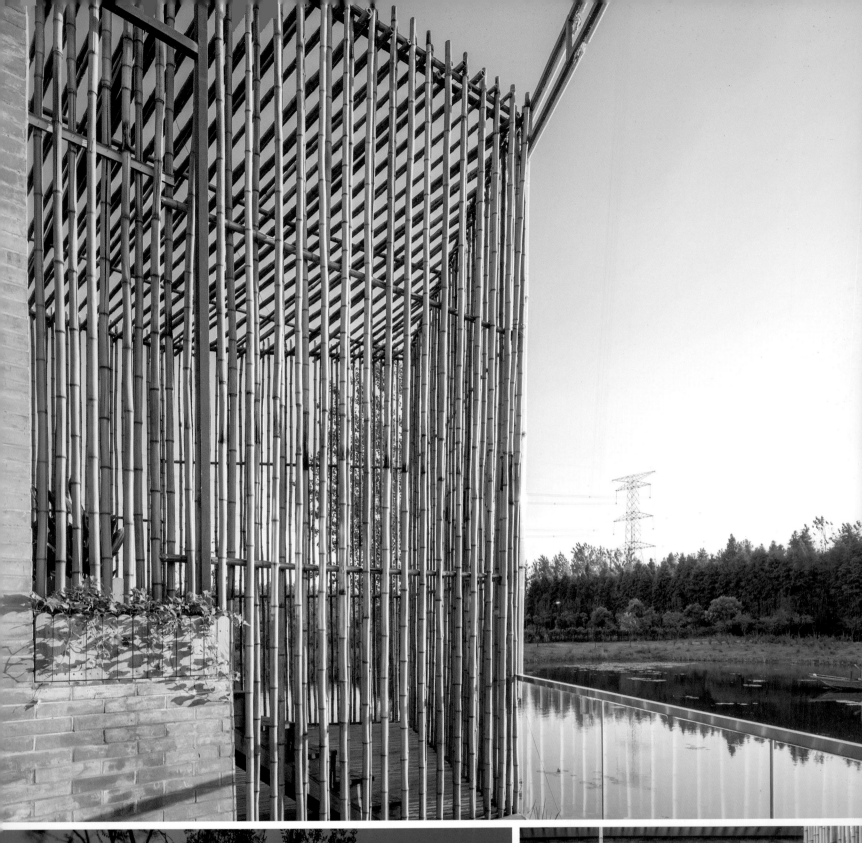

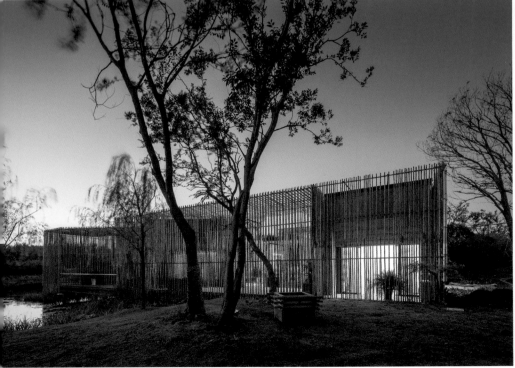

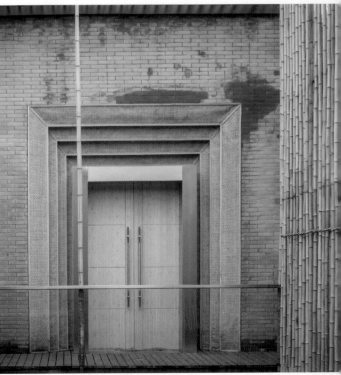

from above to below, from left to right: detail of the façade,
exterior view, entrance door

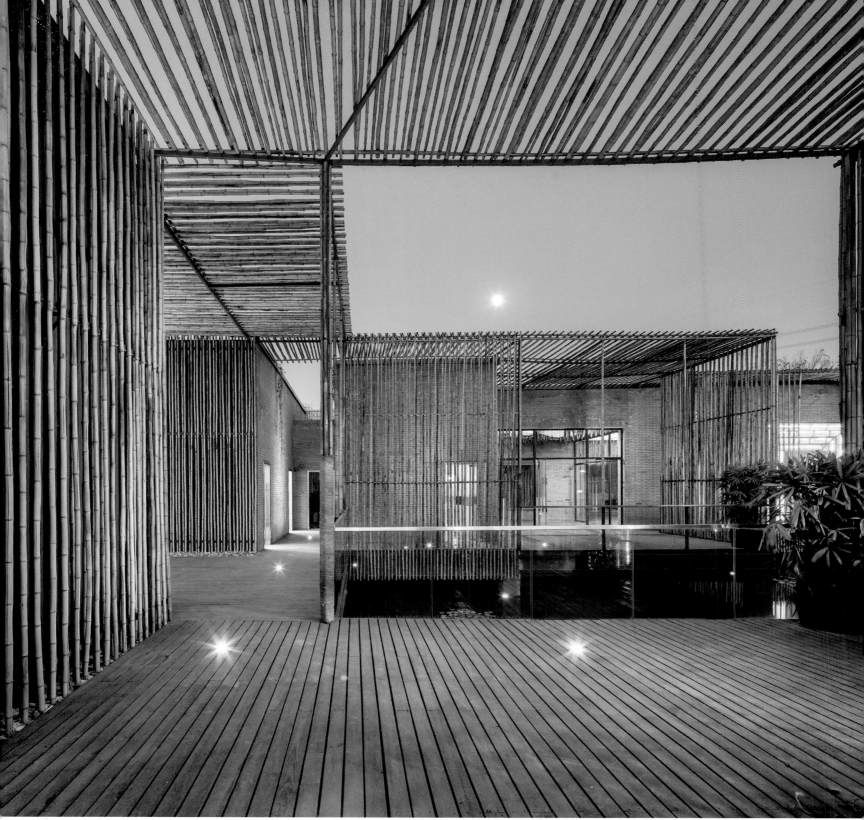

atrium

Bamboo Courtyard

Yangzhou, China

Architect: Wei Sun, HWCD
Location: ShiQiao garden, Yangzhou, Jiangsu, China
Client: construction bureau of the economy and technology development
Year of completion: 2012
Area: 400 sqm
Type of retreat: yoga retreat

In the middle of the lush ShiQiac garden is a humble tea house embracing traditional Chinese garden fundamentals and blending into the natural environment. The focal point of the tea house is the courtyard, which uses bamboo to create an interesting play of vertical and horizontal lines. In some spaces, the vertical and horizontal elements intensify to form a psychedelic perspective,

evoking a profound sensory perception. Traditionally, Yangzhou courtyards are formed with inward facing pavilions, creating an internal landscape space. Inspired by this, the bamboo courtyard was designed from a basic square footprint, fragmented into small spaces to create an internal landscape area.

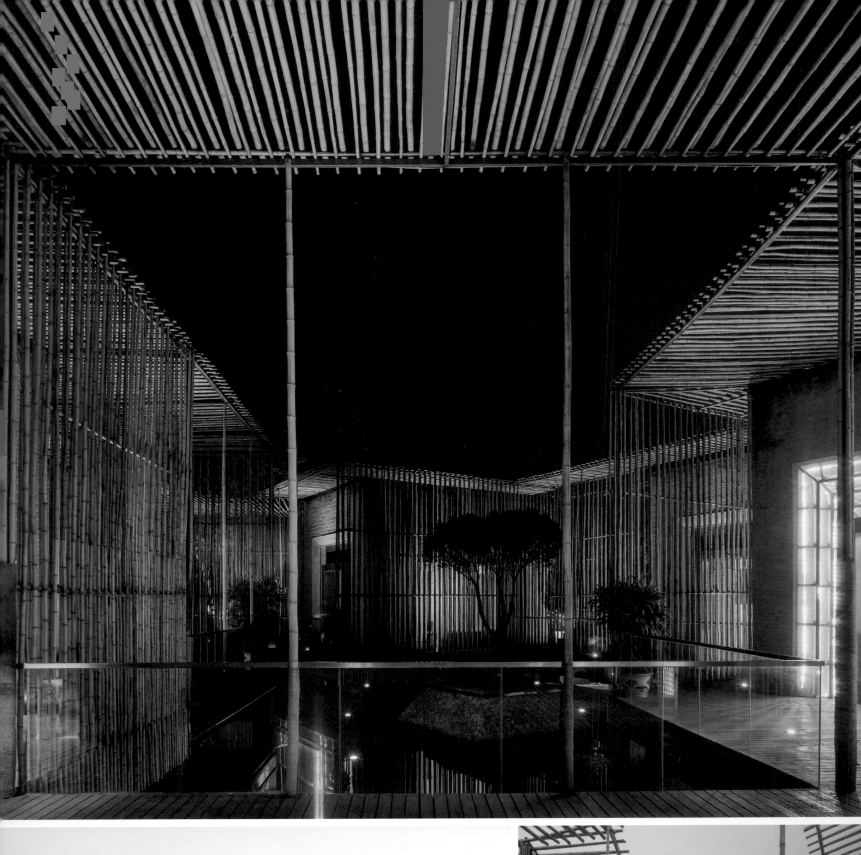

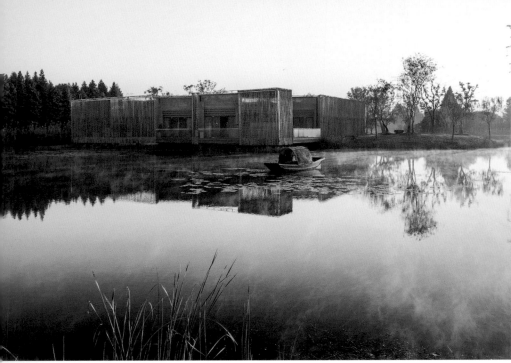

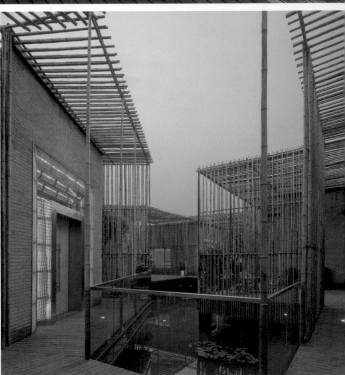

from above to below, from left to right: outdoor area, lake view, entrance area

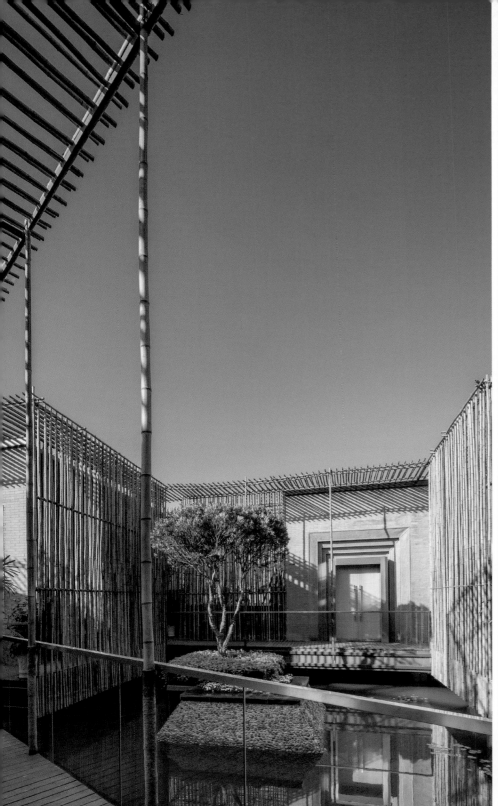

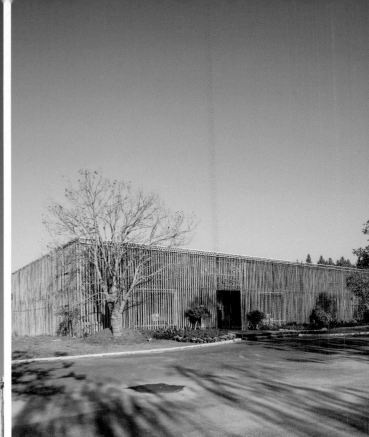

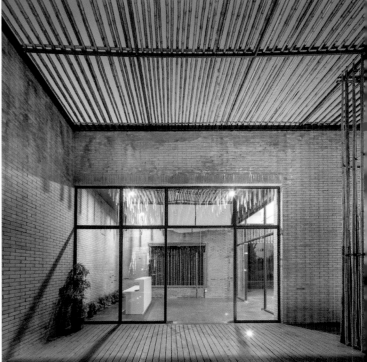

from left to right, from above to below: entrance area, reception, floor plan

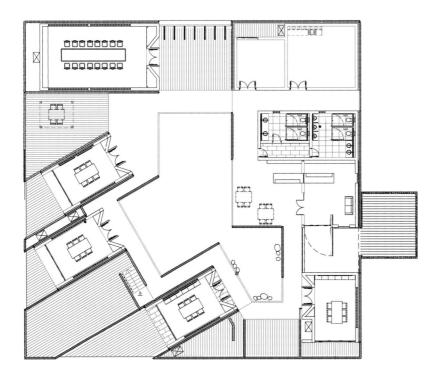

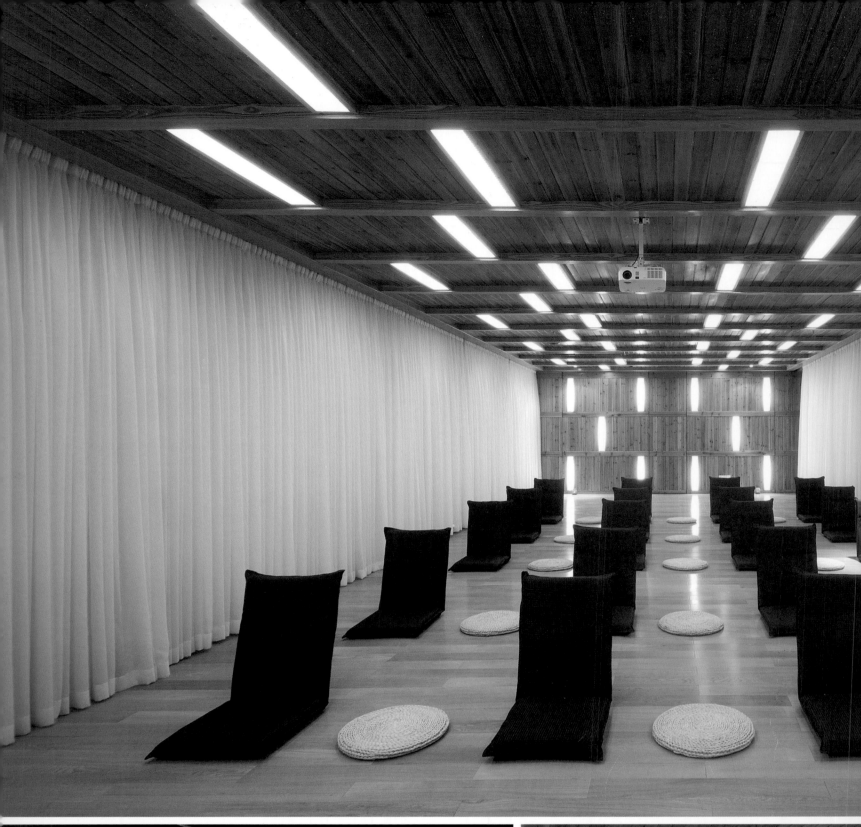

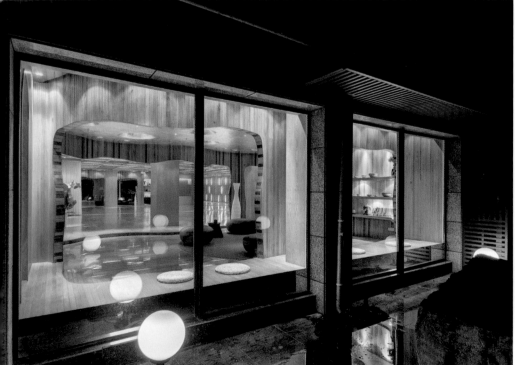

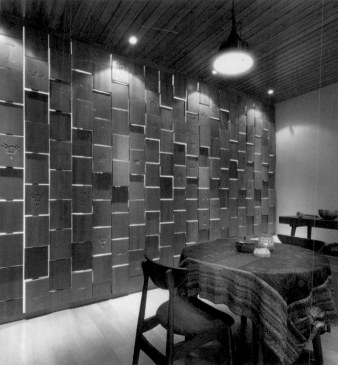

from above to below, from left to right: yoga studio, exterior view, bar

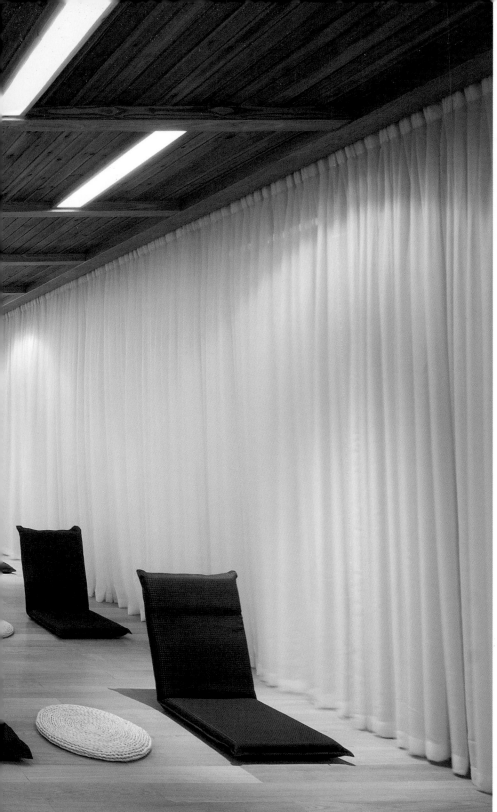

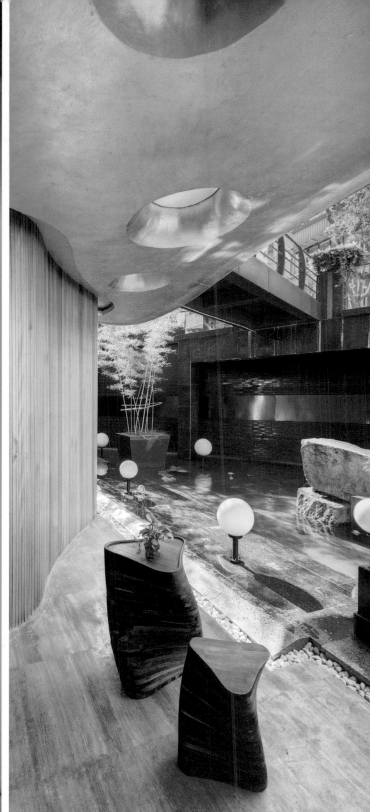

courtyard

One Taste Holistic Health

Hangzhou, China

Architect: CROX International
Location: 8-1-1 Siyi Street, Xihu, Shangcheng District, Hangzhou City, Zhejiang, China
Year of completion: 2012
Area: 360 sqm
Type of retreat: yoga studio

One Taste Holistic Health Club is located in this piece of heaven on earth between Hangzhou city's Chenghuang Temple and the West Lake. It is China's first club that focuses on the healing of minds. With a concern for the wellbeing of society, One Taste strives for spiritual enlightenment and has pioneered an open forum for re-unification with a journey back to the heart. Avant-garde architect Tsung-Jen Lin has incorporated western holism with eastern serenity to create a plane of Zen for spiritual awakening. It is a location to escape to, with a view of the West Lake from the Chenghuang Temple, high up on the mountains, where mist and haze whisper in an individua rhythm in tune with a hymn to nature.

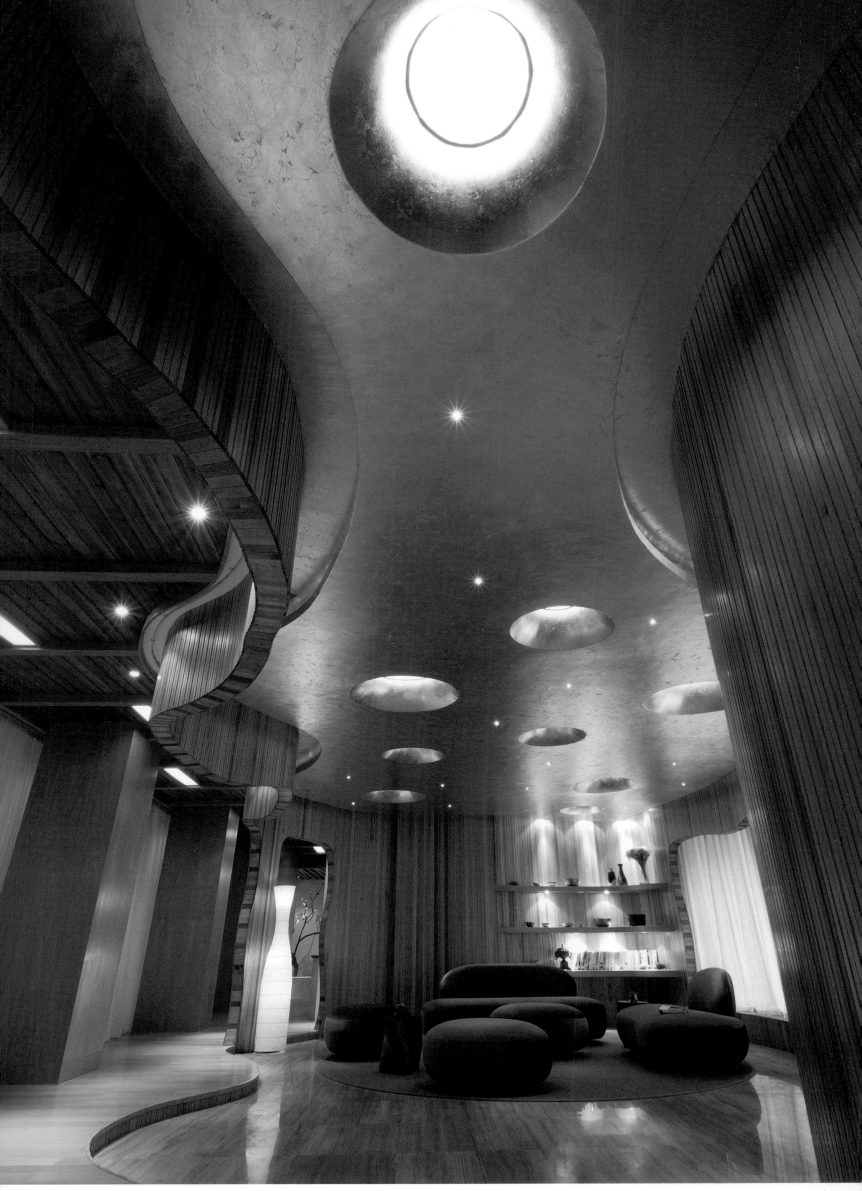

lounge area

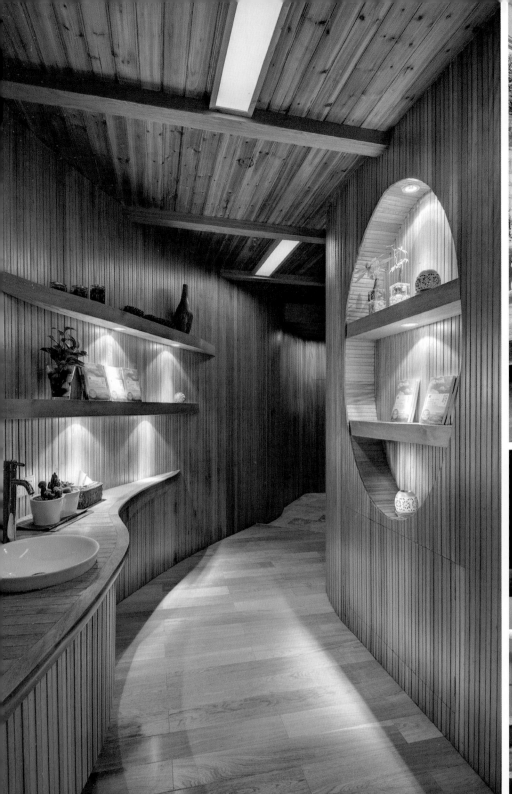

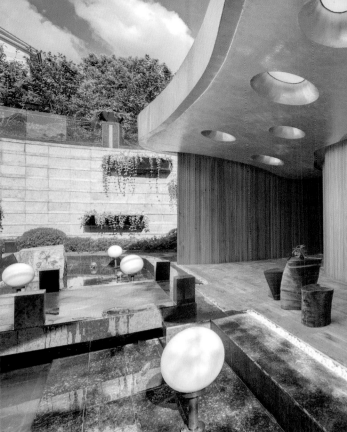

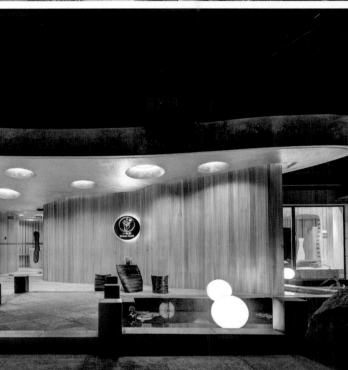

from left to right, from above to below: bathroom, garden at daytime, garden at night, floor plan

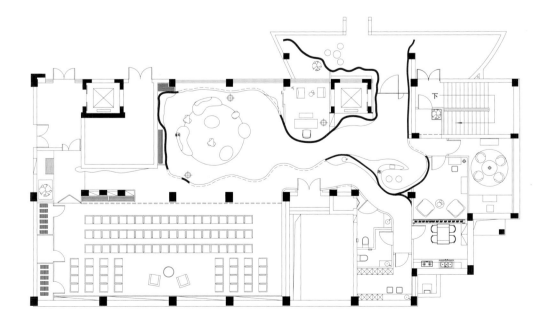

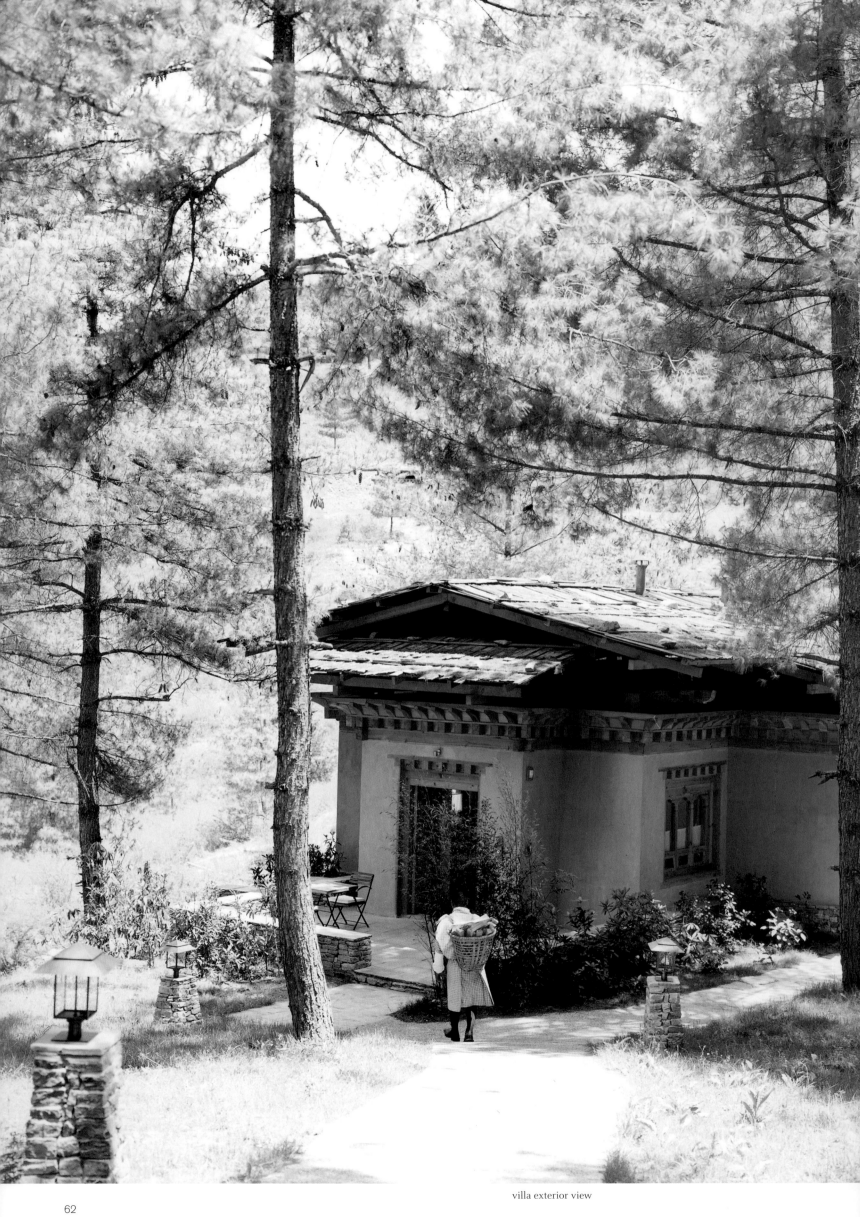

villa exterior view

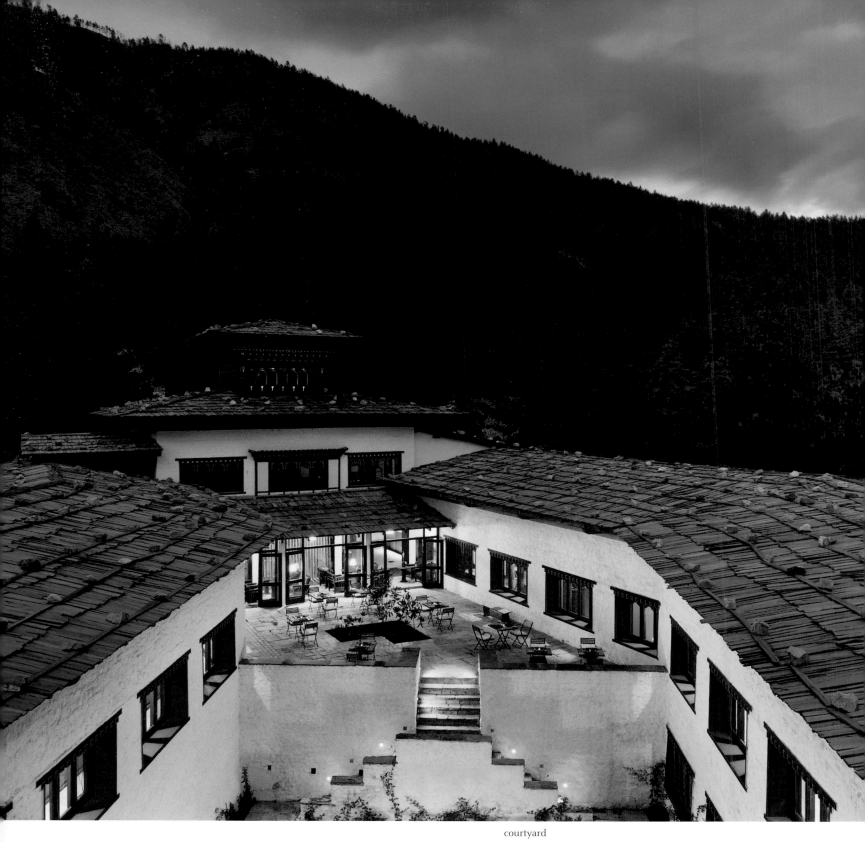

courtyard

Uma by COMO

Paro, Bhutan

Architect: Cheong Yew Kuan
Year of completion: 2004
Type of retreat: spiritual retreat

Uma Paro offers luxury in the heart of Bhutan. Hotel guests enjoy sweeping views of the pristine Himalayas from the 38-acre estate, comprising a mere twenty rooms and nine mansions with a design that is a subtle fusion of indigenous style, and fresh, clean-lined modernism. But Uma Paro also offers adventure. The town of Paro, Bhutan's main cultural hub, is nearby. Hiking, mountain biking and overnight luxury camping trips are all available. Guests can later recoup and indulge in vital holistic therapies at COMO Shambhala Retreat, and dine in style at the Bukhari restaurant, where local Bhutanese produce is blended with Indian cuisine.

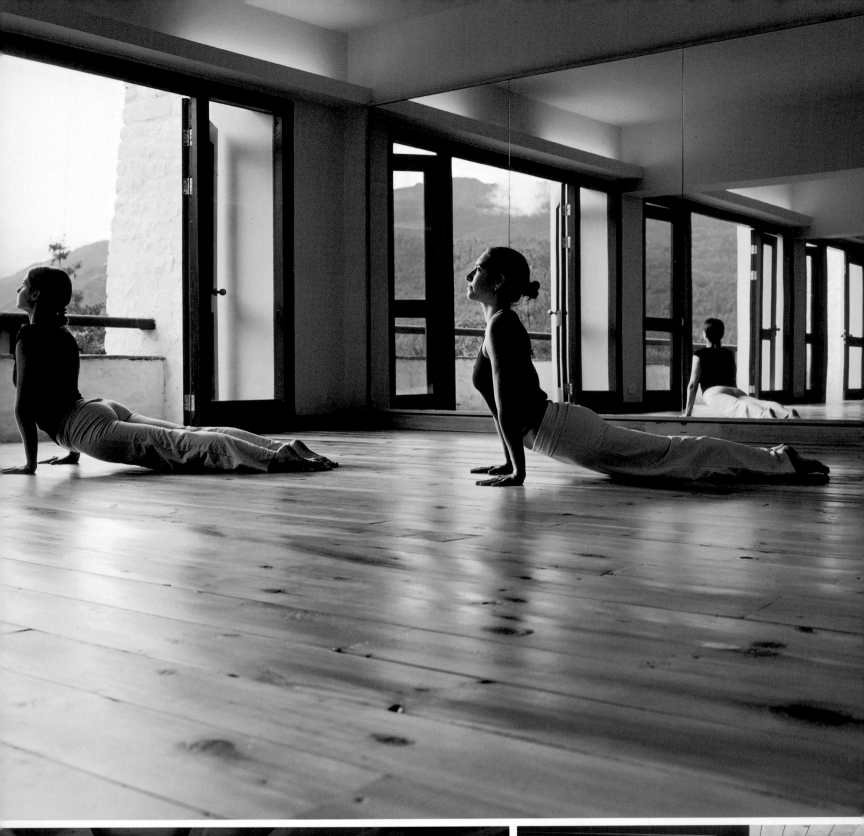

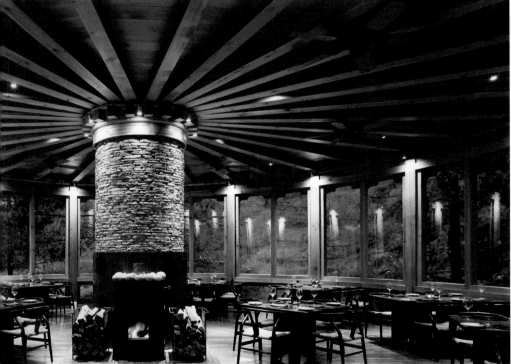

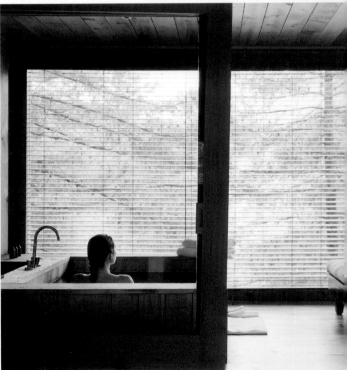

from above to below, from left to right: yoga studio,
restaurant, stone bath house

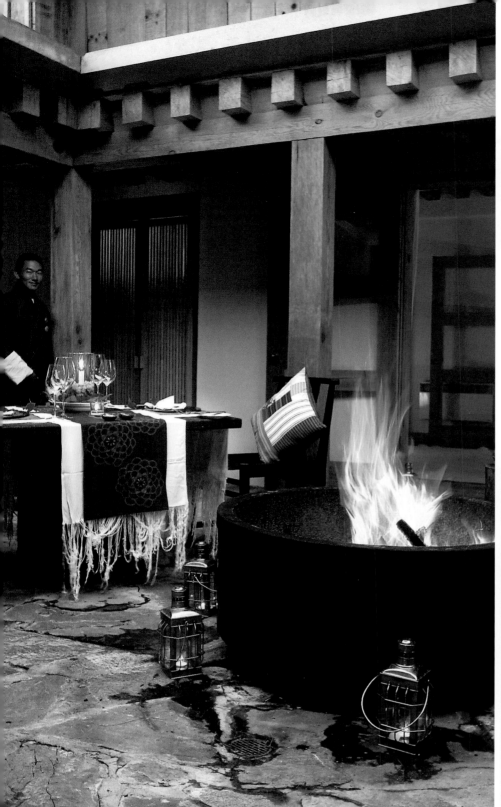
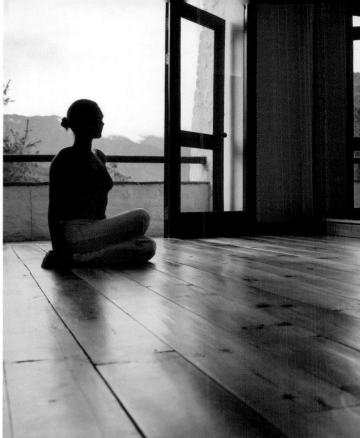
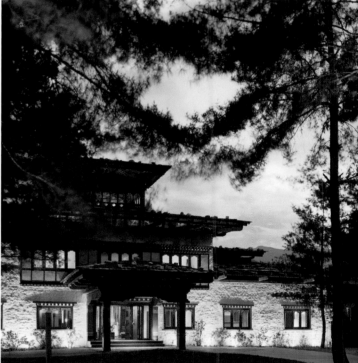
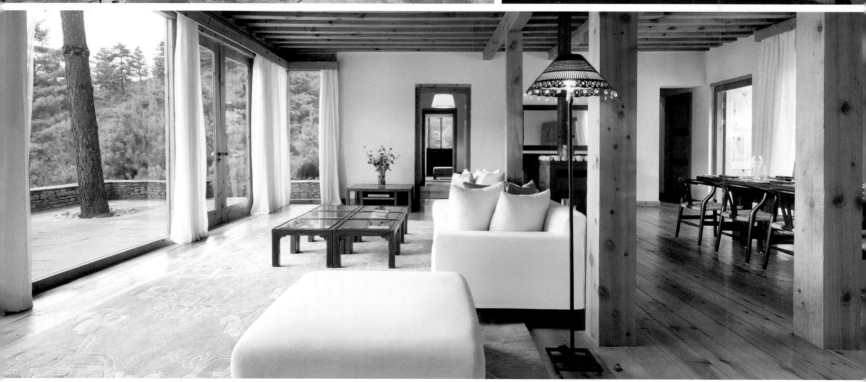

from left to right, from above to below: courtyard view, yoga
studio, entrance, villa living room

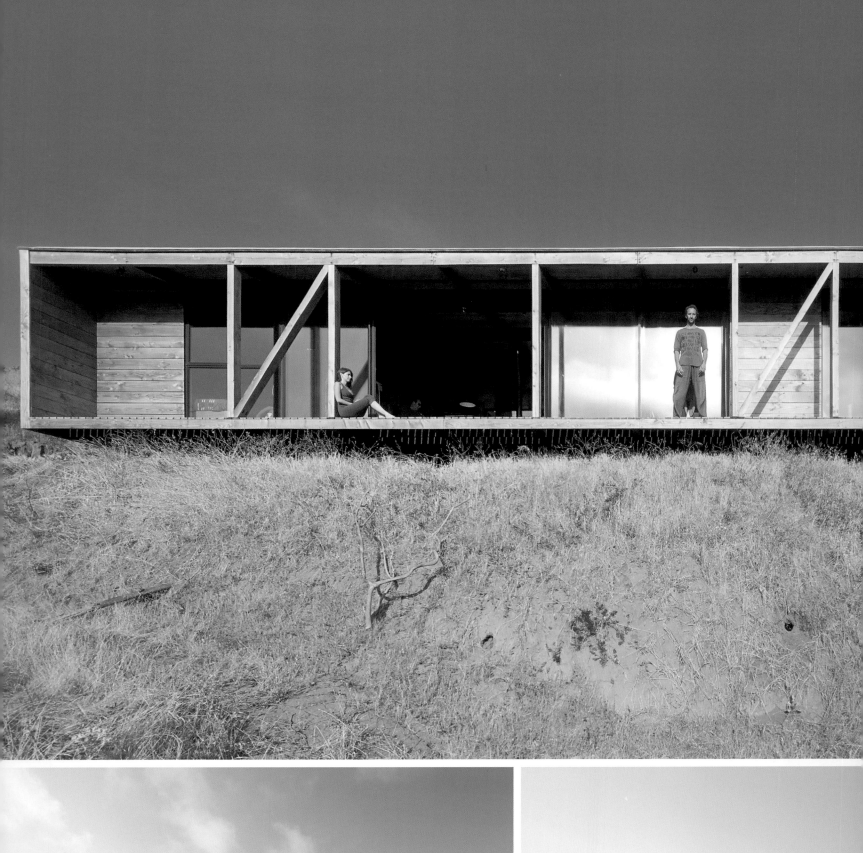

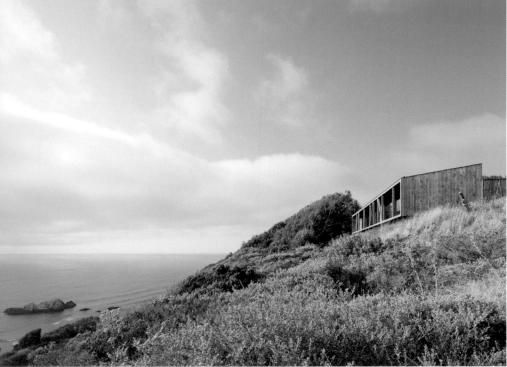

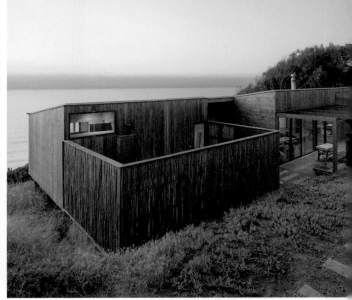

from above to below, from left to right: exterior view, overview, outdoor area

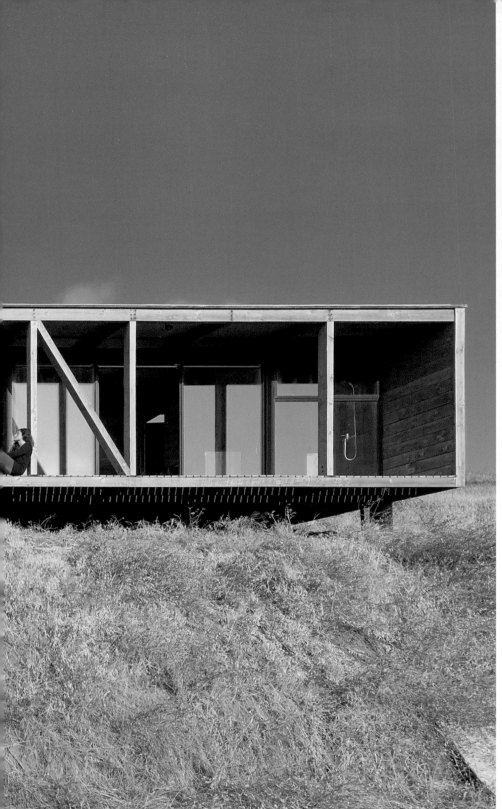

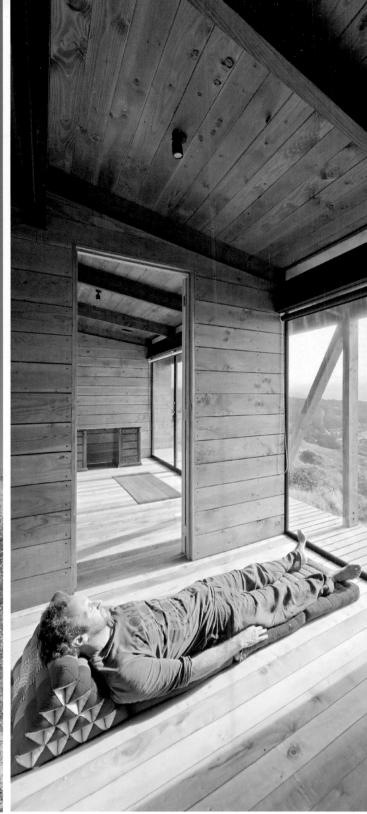

meditation

Yoga House
Matanzas, Chile

Architect: WMR Arquitectos
Location: Matanzas, Navidad, Libertador General Bernardo O'Higgins Region, Chile
Year of completion: 2011
Area: 140 sqm
Type of retreat: private house

Set on the mountainside of Matanzas beach, overlooking the bay. The primary design intention was to integrate the building within the powerful landscape slope and to derive its poetics from the qualities of its surroundings. The design embeds the house in the hill to generate a back yard patio, exposed to the morning light, which along with the main entrance is protected from the wind. The intention was to extend the view of the sea from the back-yard

through the house. The kitchen, dining and living room are located next to the back yard in a level below the rest of the house. This allows the integration of the back yard with the house. It also shares the same materiality stone. The rest of the house is built with timber. Designed in a more cozy and intimate manner, the yoga room connects the living room with both bedrooms.

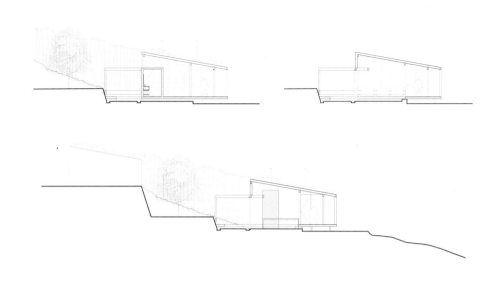

from above to below: sections, panorama view

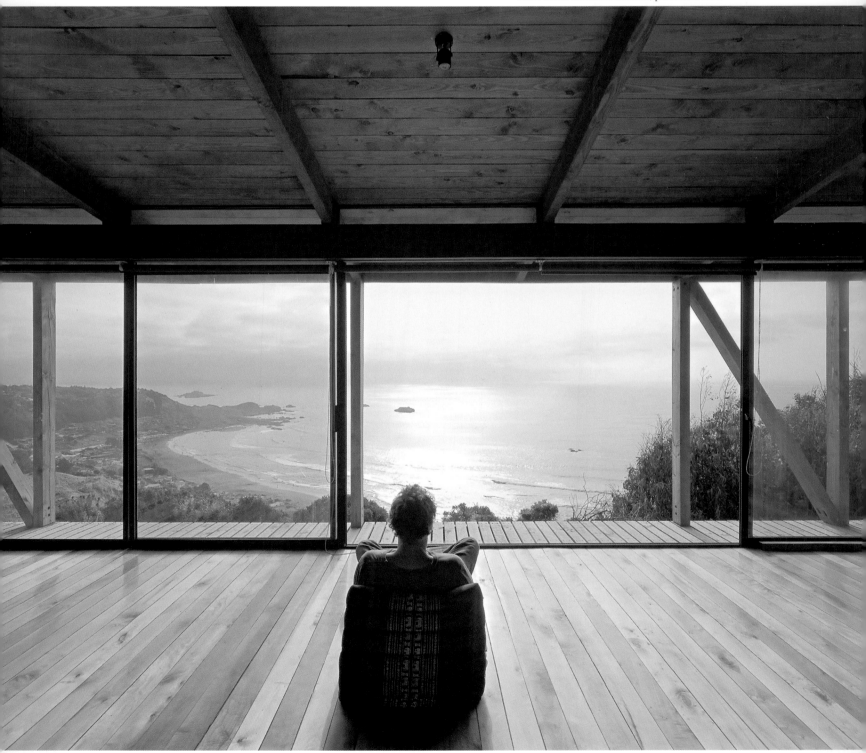

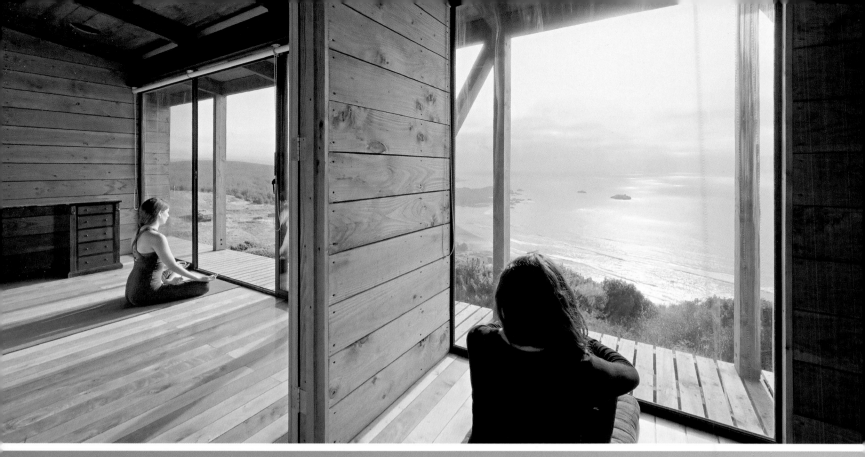

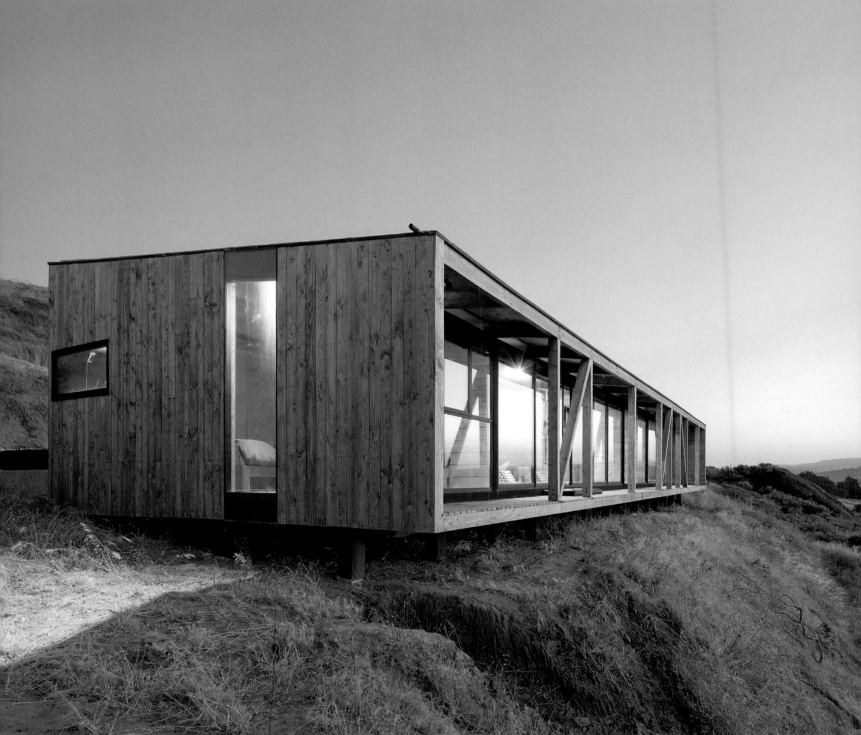

from above to below: people practicing yoga, exterior view

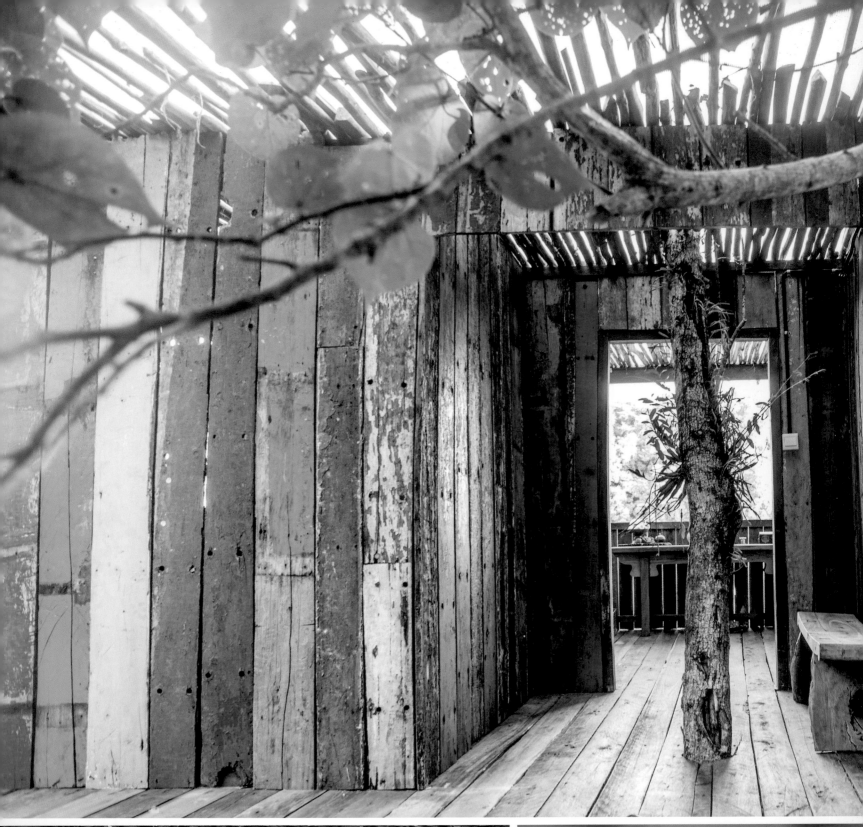

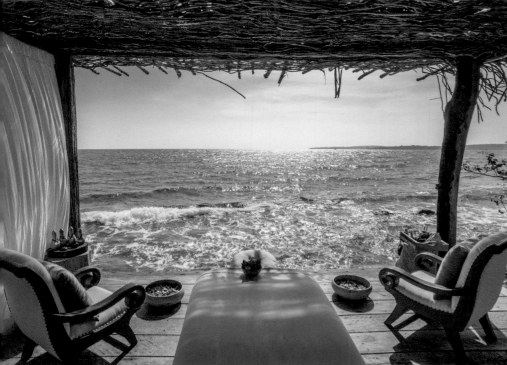

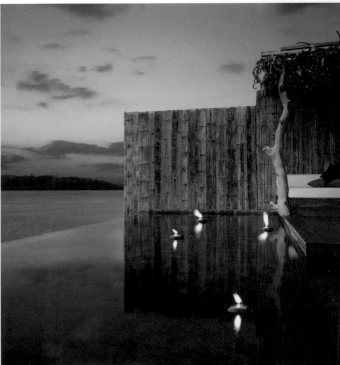

from above to below, from left to right: interior design, open spa treatment room over water, villa at night

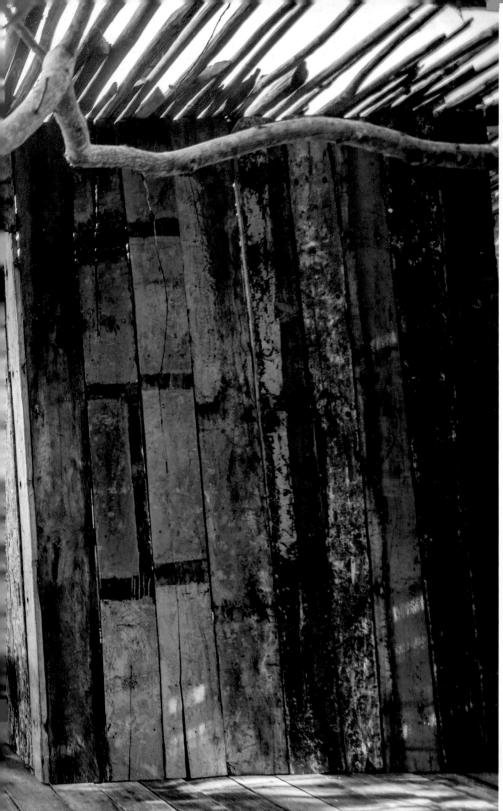

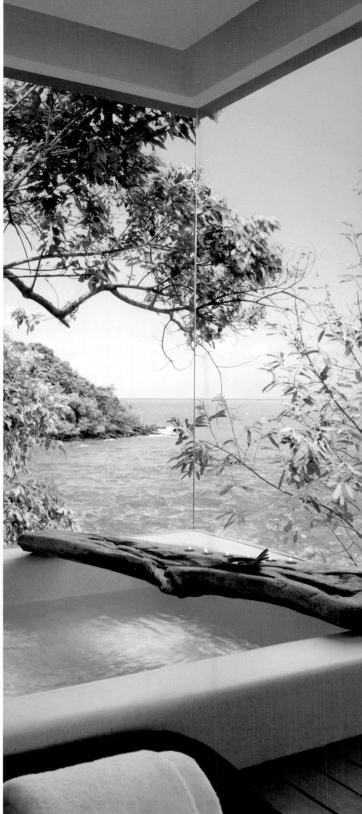

bathroom

Song Saa Private Island

Koh Rong, Cambodia

Architect:
Melita Hunter & Rory Hunter
Location: Koh Ouen,
Koh Rong, Cambodia
Year of completion: 2012
Area: 40,000 sqm
Type of retreat: luxury
private island resort

The Robinson Crusoe feeling meets upscale barefoot tourism: wild, unspoiled nature, lush tropical interior and barefoot beaches as smooth as satin. There, in the Cambodian archipelago of Koh Rong in the Gulf of Thailand, is the idyllic luxury hideaway Song Saa Private Island. The exclusive resort surrounded by nature consists of twenty-seven private mansions extending over the islands of Koh Ouen and Koh Bong, connected only by a suspension bridge. The treatments in the holistic tradition of Buddhism are harmoniously integrated in the stay on Song Saa Private Island and enable those in search of rest the deepest relaxation and sense of wellbeing in a new affinity with the energy of life.

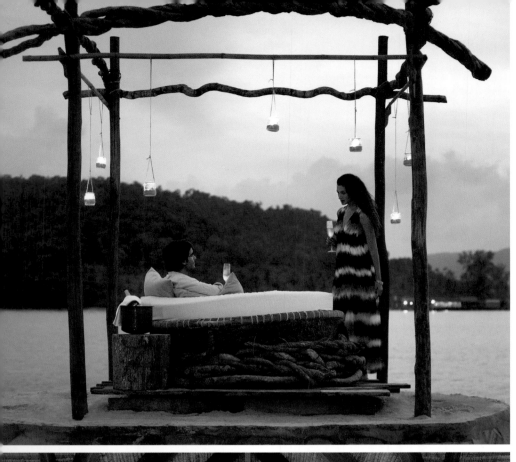

from above to below, from left to right: bar at the beach, living room, bathroom, overwater deck at sunset

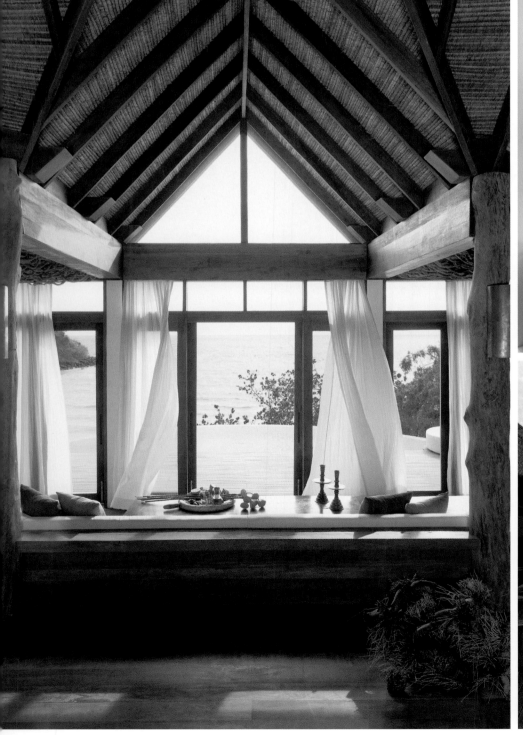

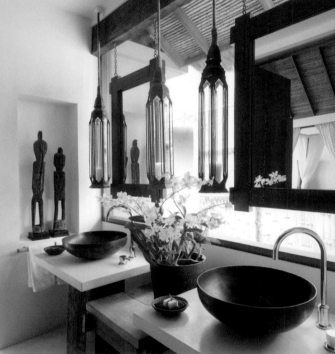

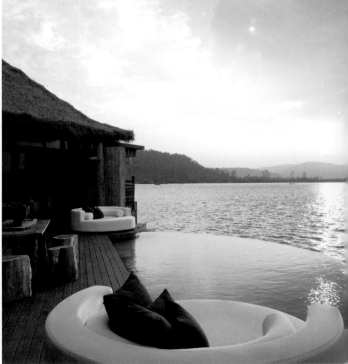

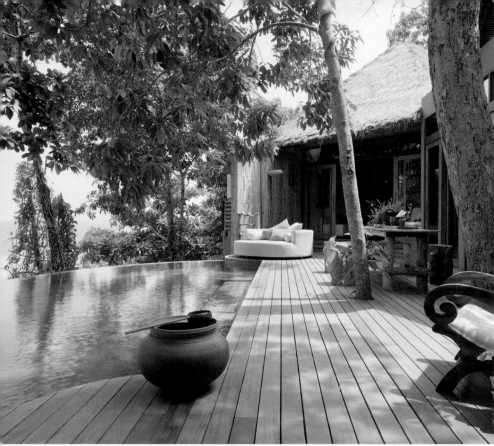
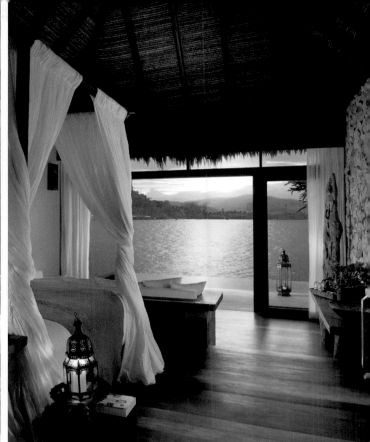
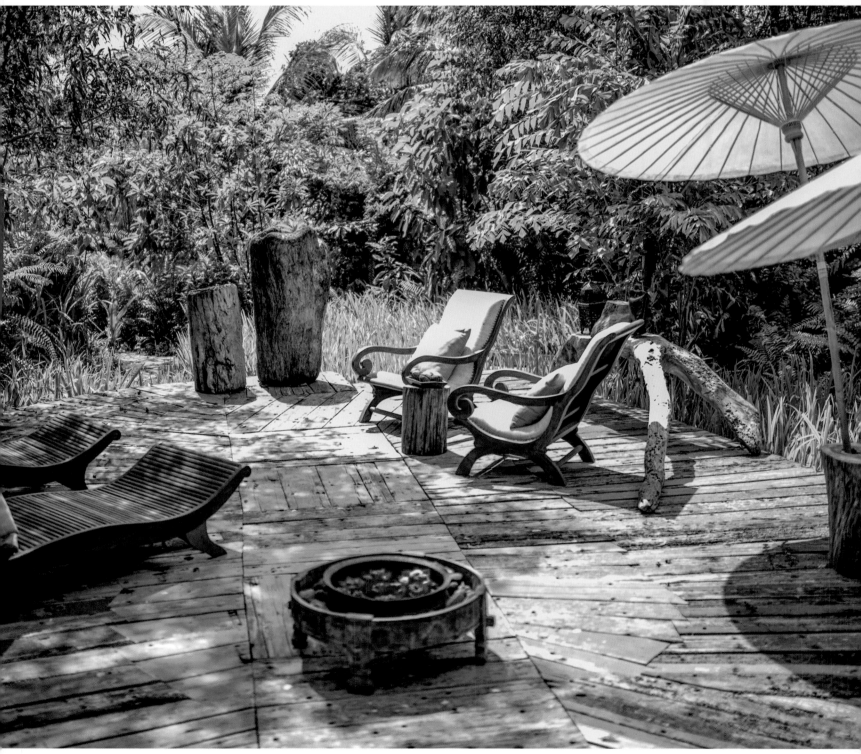

from left to right, from above to below: villa with pool,
bedroom, terrace

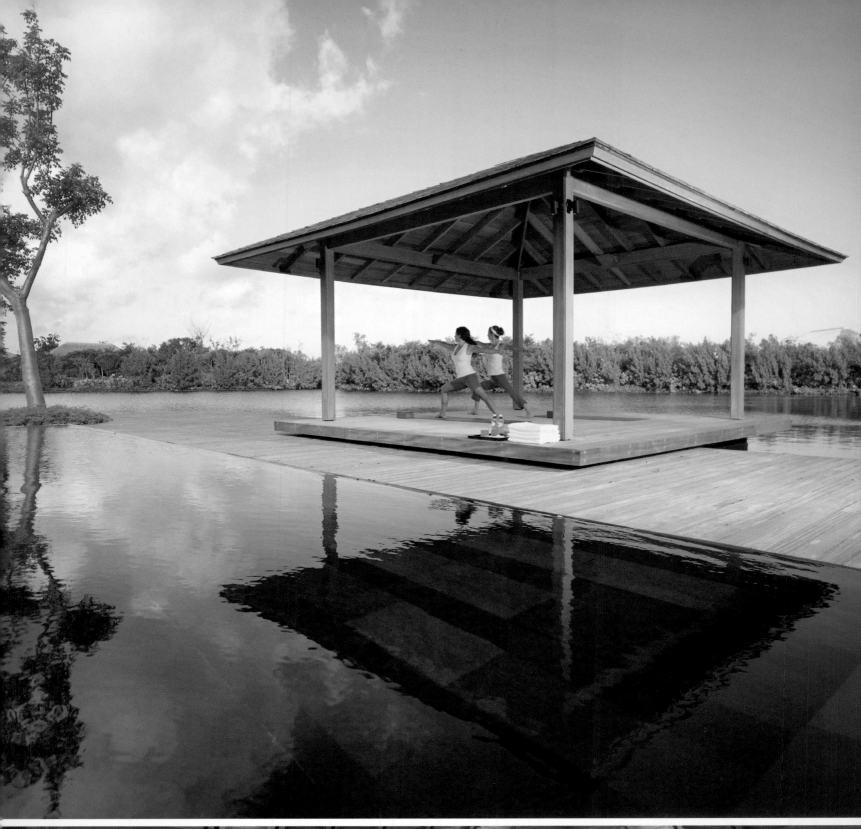

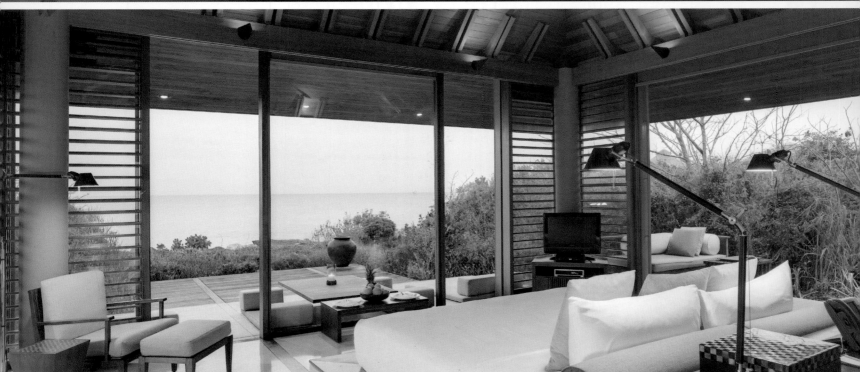

from above to below: yoga pavilion, interior view

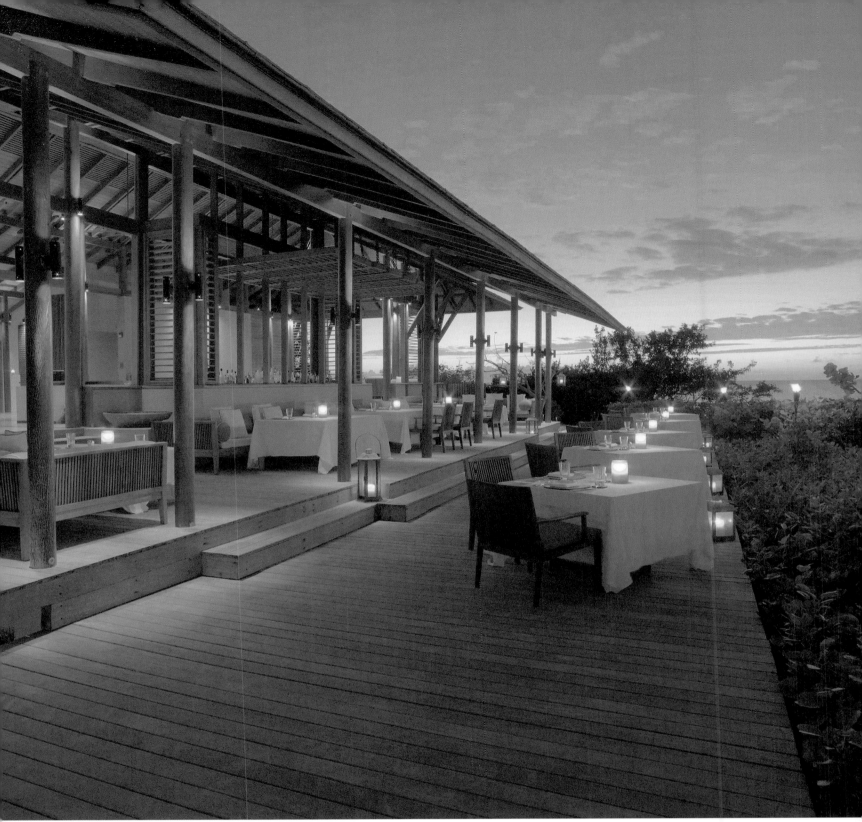

Yara beach club

Amanyara

Providenciales, Turks and Caicos Islands

Architect: Jean-Michel Gathy
Location: Providenciales, Turks and Caicos Islands, British West Indies
Year of completion: 2006
Type of retreat: resort

Set on a secluded white-sand beach, Amanyara enjoys a pristine location well removed from much of the development on the eastern side of the island of Providenciales. The resort is open to the elements – the sun and its reflection off the water, the sea breeze and the sights and sounds of the ocean. Entry to the resort is through a large reception pavilion that opens onto a central reflection pond. Amanyara offers 36 timber-shingled guest pavilions as well as a selection of exclusive mansions. Surrounded by mahogany trees, the pond is framed on one side by the Library and Gallery, and on the other side by the Restaurant and Bar. The circular Bar offers a dramatically soaring roof and sea views fronted by the 50-meter main swimming pool and sun deck.

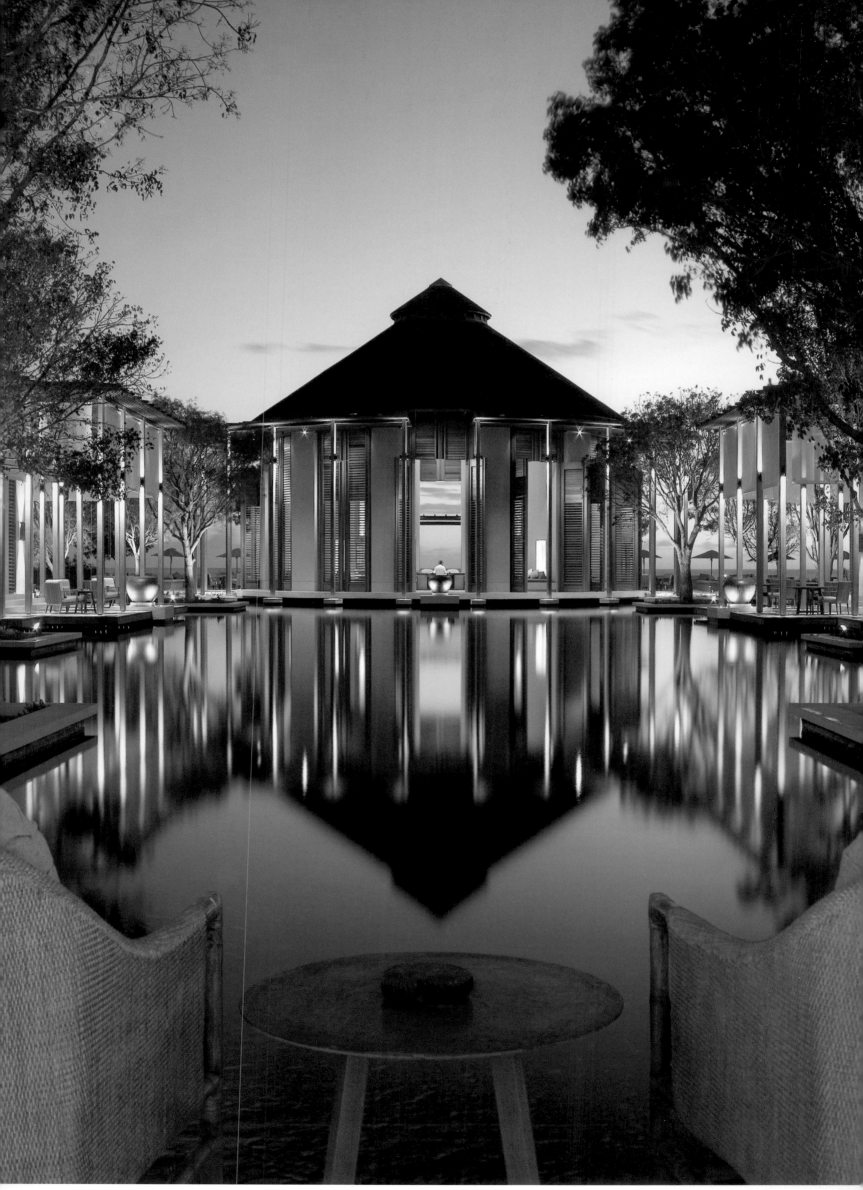

grand reflecting pond

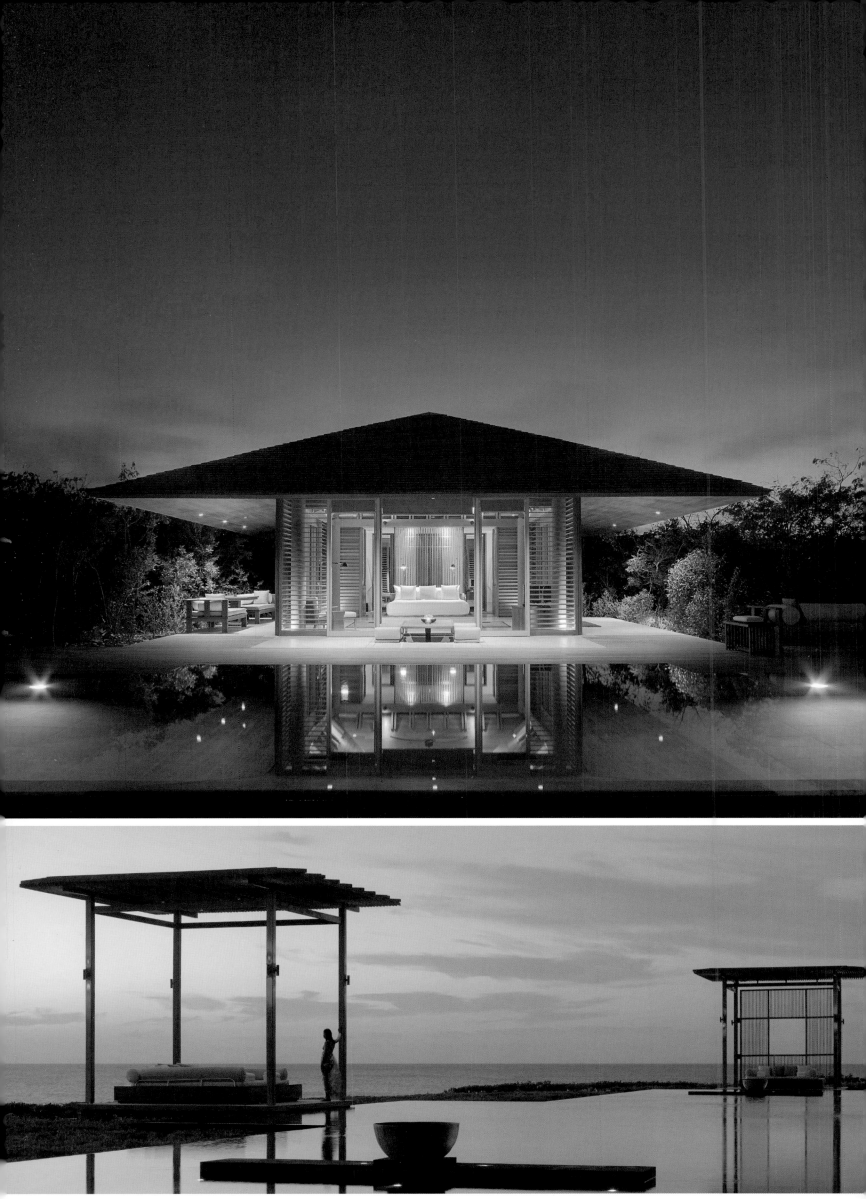

from above to below: pool pavilion, pool with ocean view

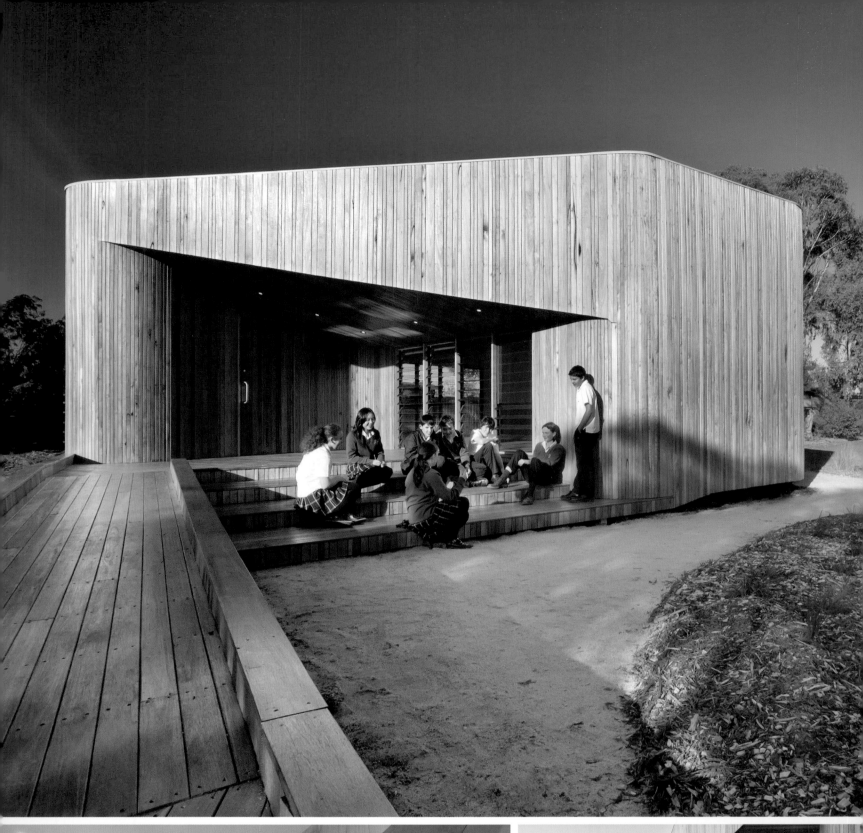

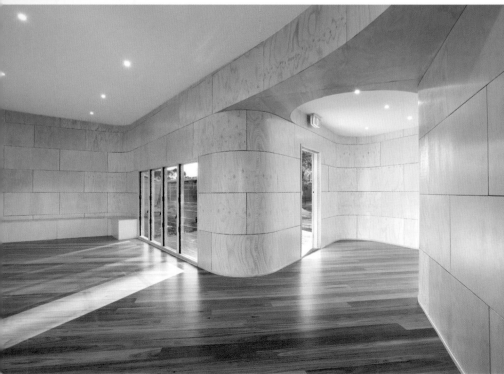

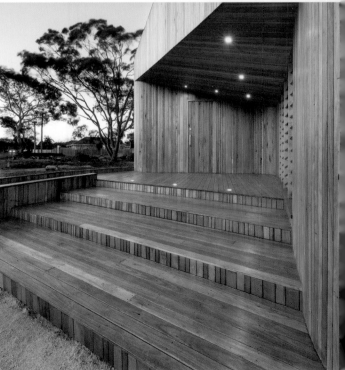

from above to below, from left to right: exterior view, interior
view, entrance

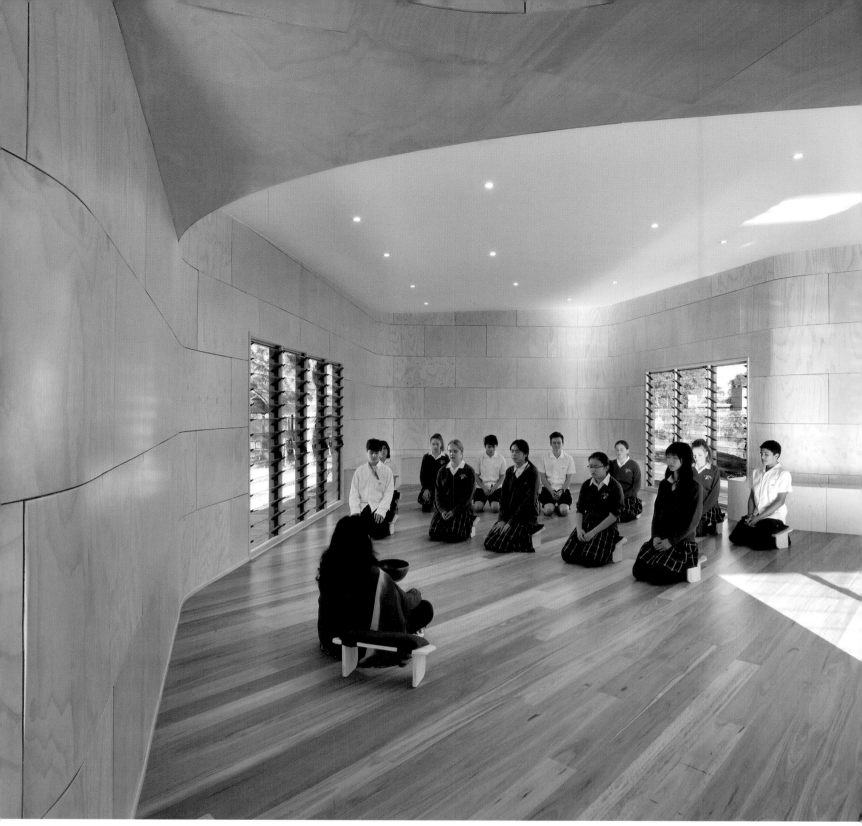

Bentleigh Secondary College

Melbourne, Australia

Architect: dwp|suters architecture + interior design
Location: Vivian Street, East Bentleigh, Melbourne, VIC 3165, Australia
Year of completion: 2013
Area: 109 sqm
Type of retreat: education & mindful meditation

The Meditation and Indigenous Cultural Centre was conceived to fill three primary roles: to provide a space for the school's mindfulness meditation program; educate students about sustainable design; and be a focus for the school's indigenous curriculum. All students learn the art of mindfulness meditation which helps them to unclutter their minds, respond skilfully to emotions and focus calmly on the present. The design creates a warm uniform space that reflects the contrasting nature of our inner and outer self through materiality and form. In essence the inside of the building will maintain its 'youthful' appearance whilst the external will develop and mature with age.

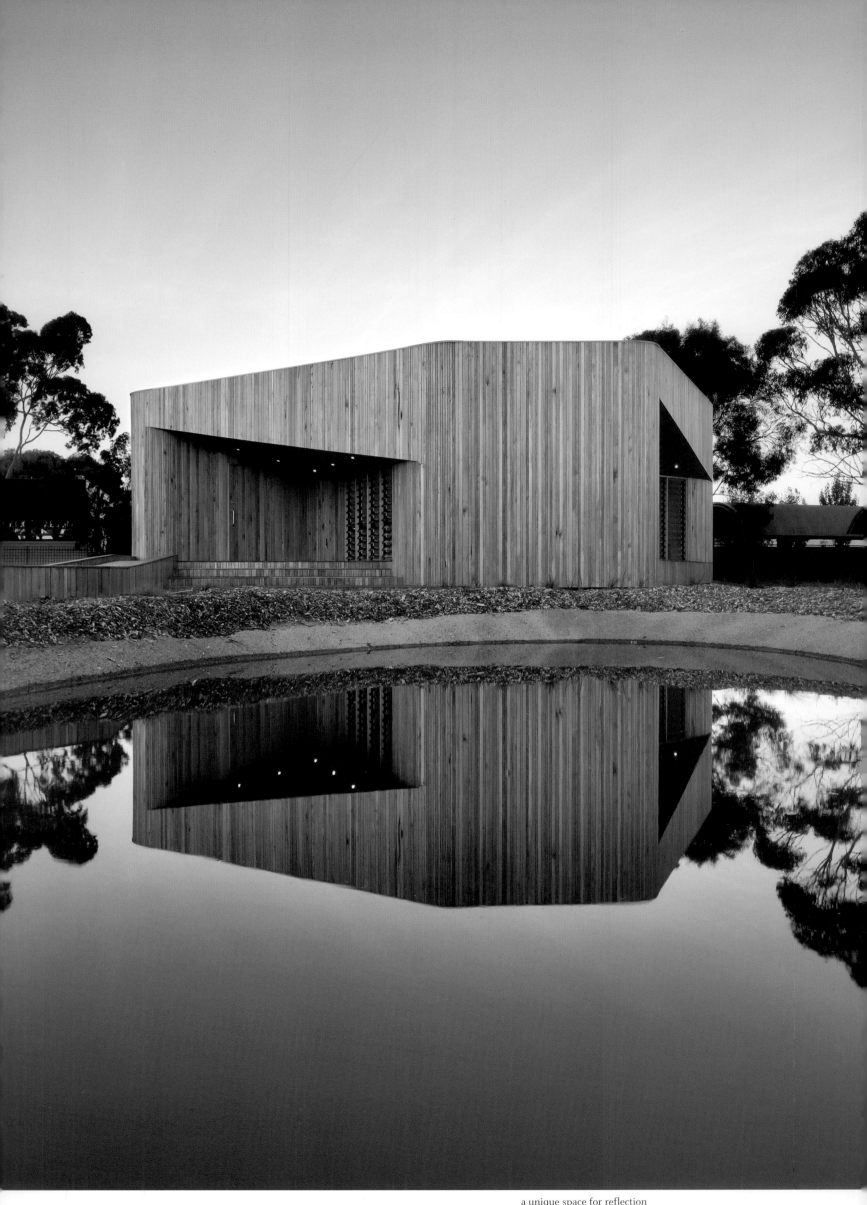

a unique space for reflection

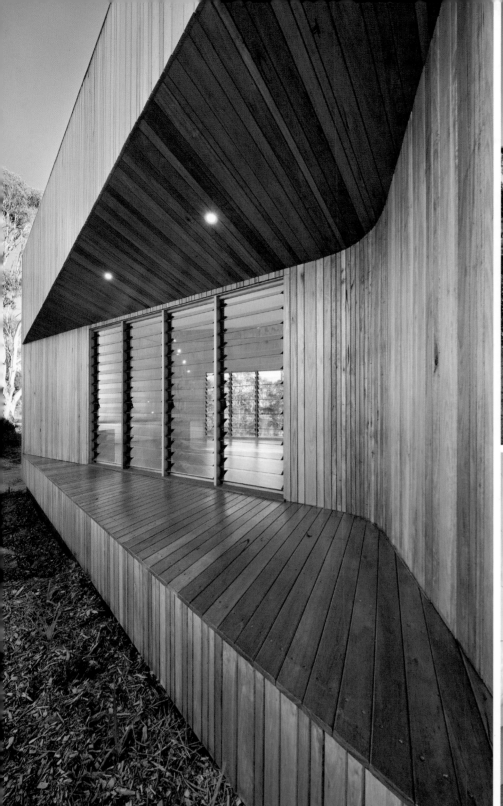
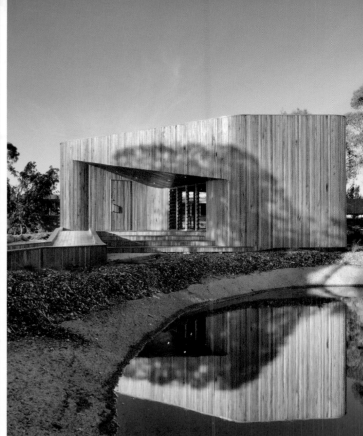
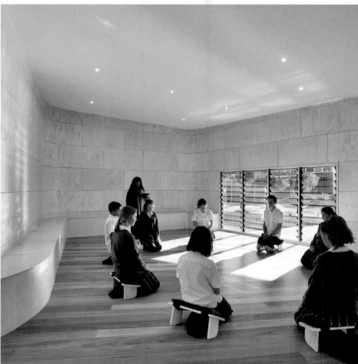

from left to right, from above to below: large awnings ensure solar heat gain, exterior view, children practicing meditation, site plan

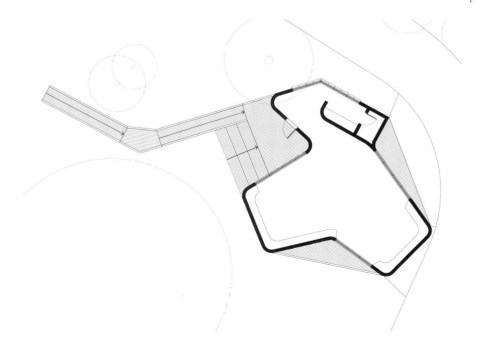

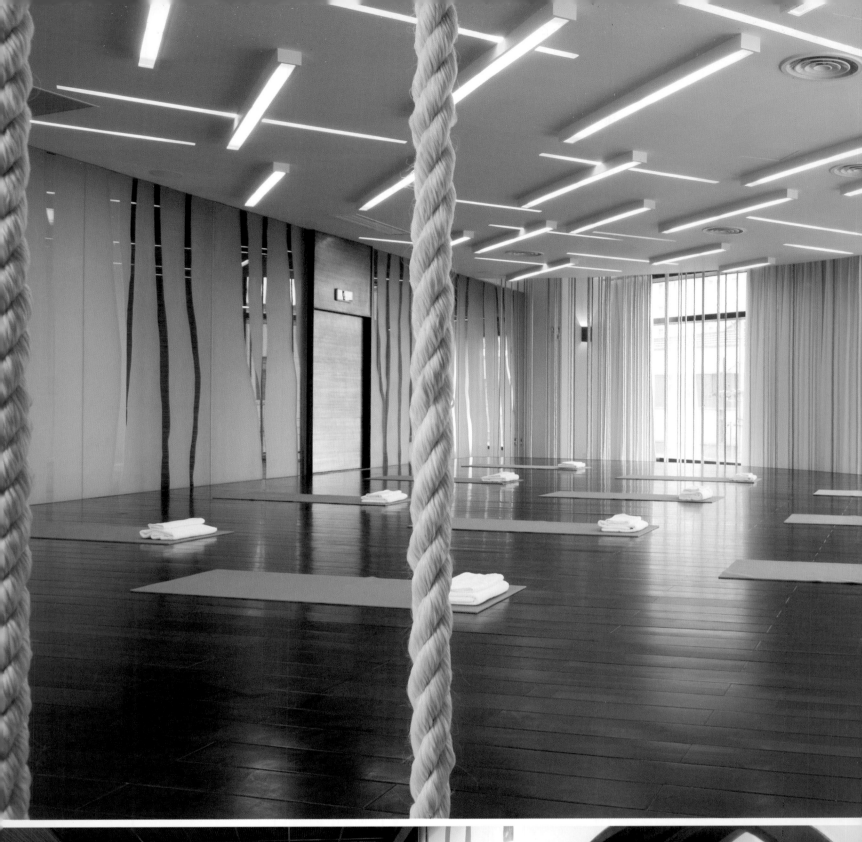

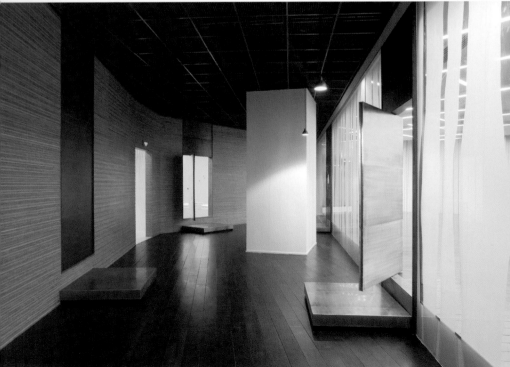

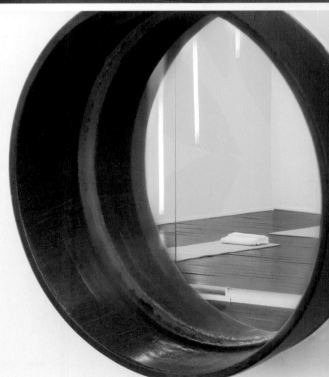

from above to below, from left to right: yoga studio, hall, detail of the wall

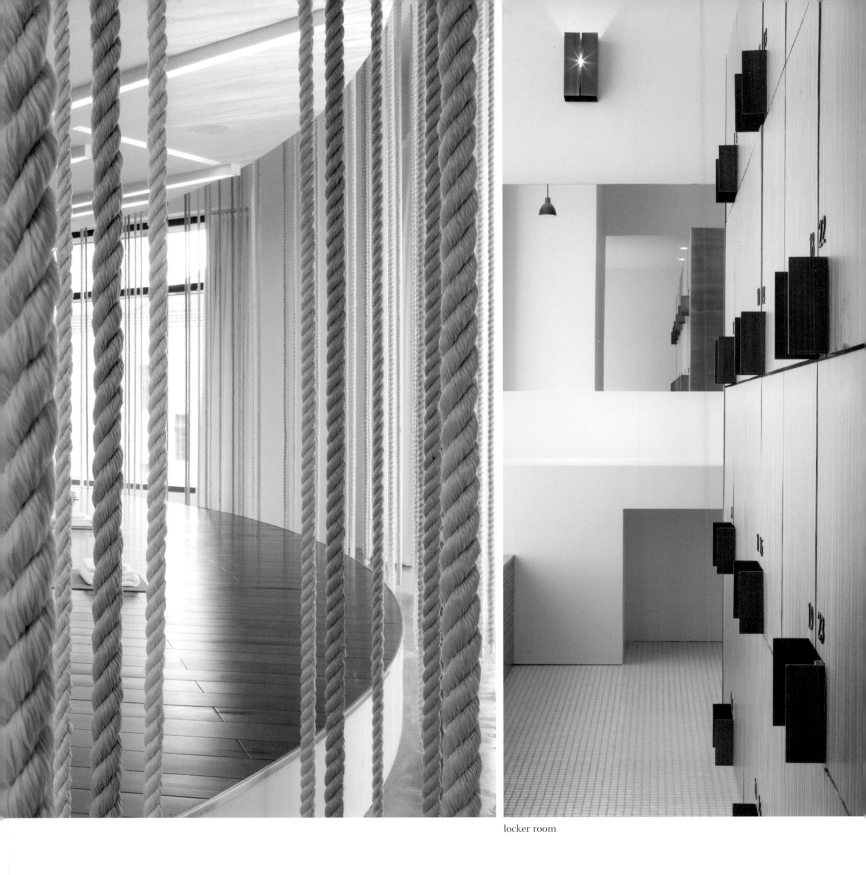

locker room

The Voyeuristic Wall

Shanghai, China

Architect: Neri&Hu Design and Research Office
Location: 88 Yuqing Road, 200030, Shanghai, China
Year of completion: 2006
Area: 1,200 sqm
Type of retreat: health, wellness & yoga center

Y+ Yoga and Wellness Center is a 1,200 square meters extension of the original Y+ Yoga studio concept. Y+ is inarguably a primary force in augmenting the concept of lifestyle in Shanghai. The design explores the abstract concept of tranquility by creating intimate spaces for self-reflection and communal spaces for human encounters. These include rooms for cooling down, reading, chatting and meeting new people. The main yoga room is an elevated half-circular room in an abstracted forest, represented by vertically hanging ropes. More than simply a place for exercise, the environment enforces the slow-down of pace, encouraging students to relax, read, and enjoy their yoga as something more than a path towards fitness.

83

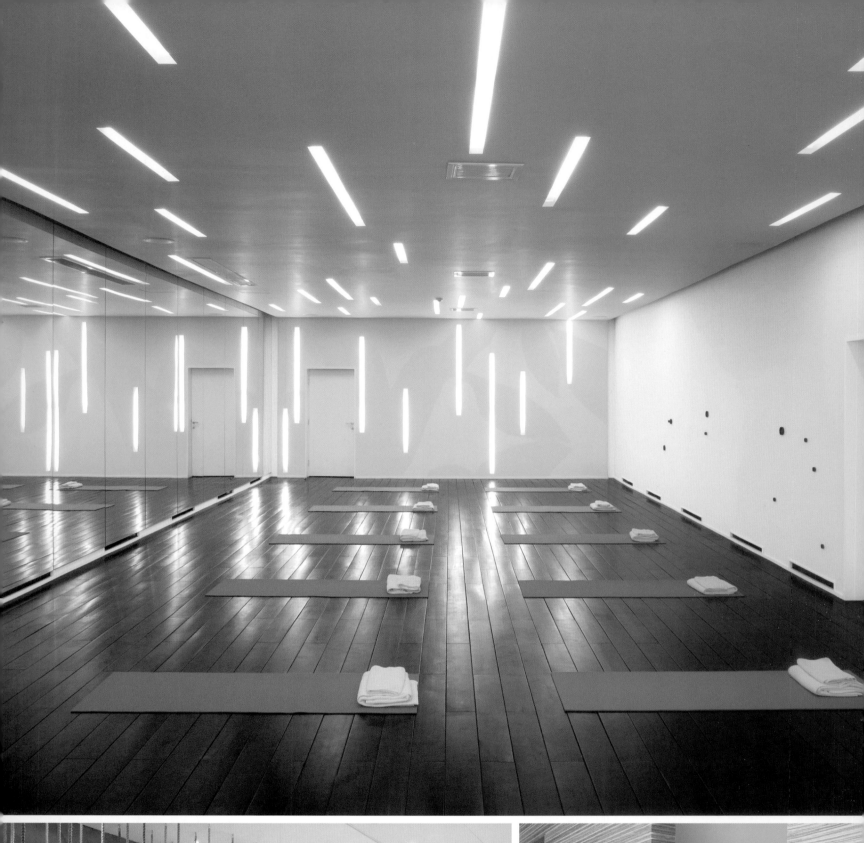

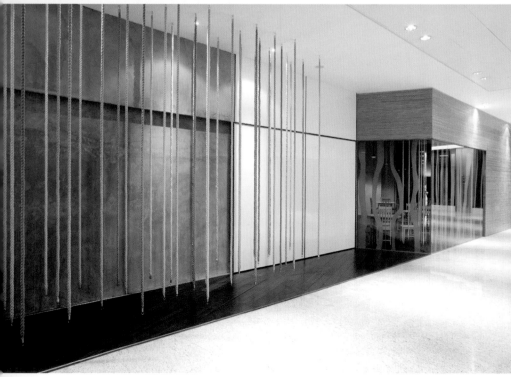

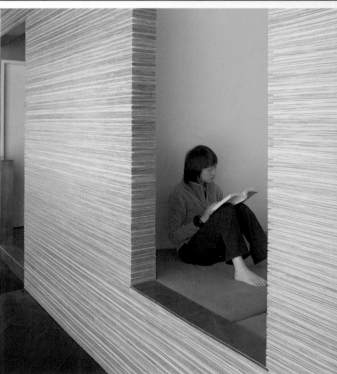

from above to below, from left to right: yoga studio, reception, chill-out area

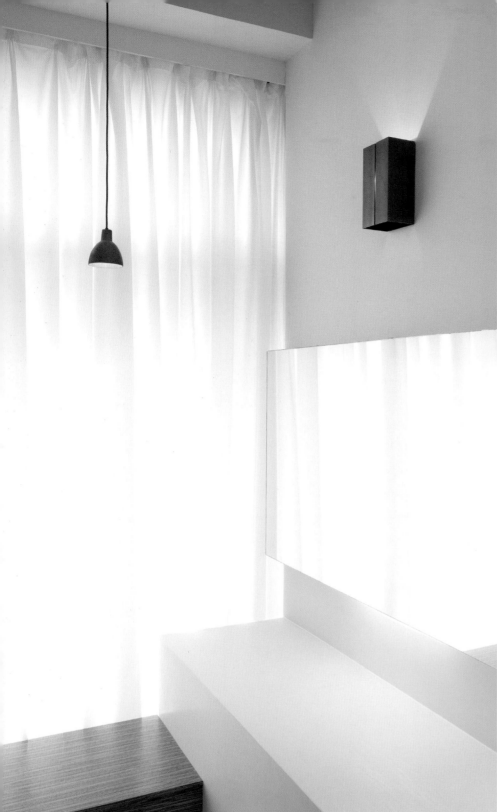

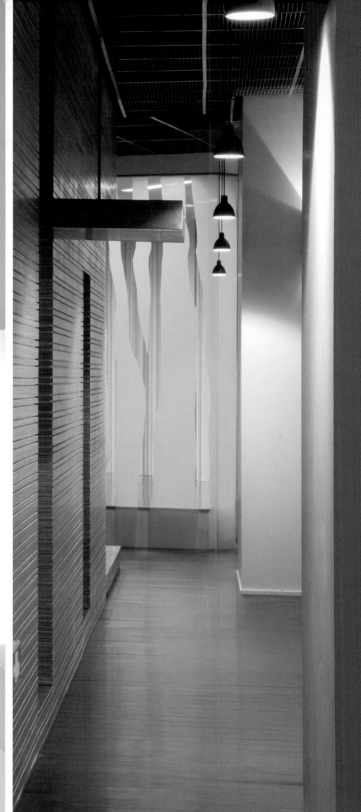

from left to right, from above to below: interior view, entrance area, floor plan

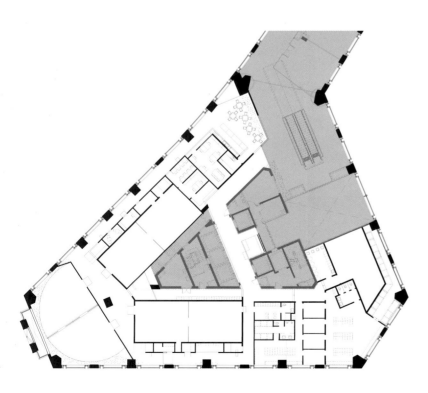

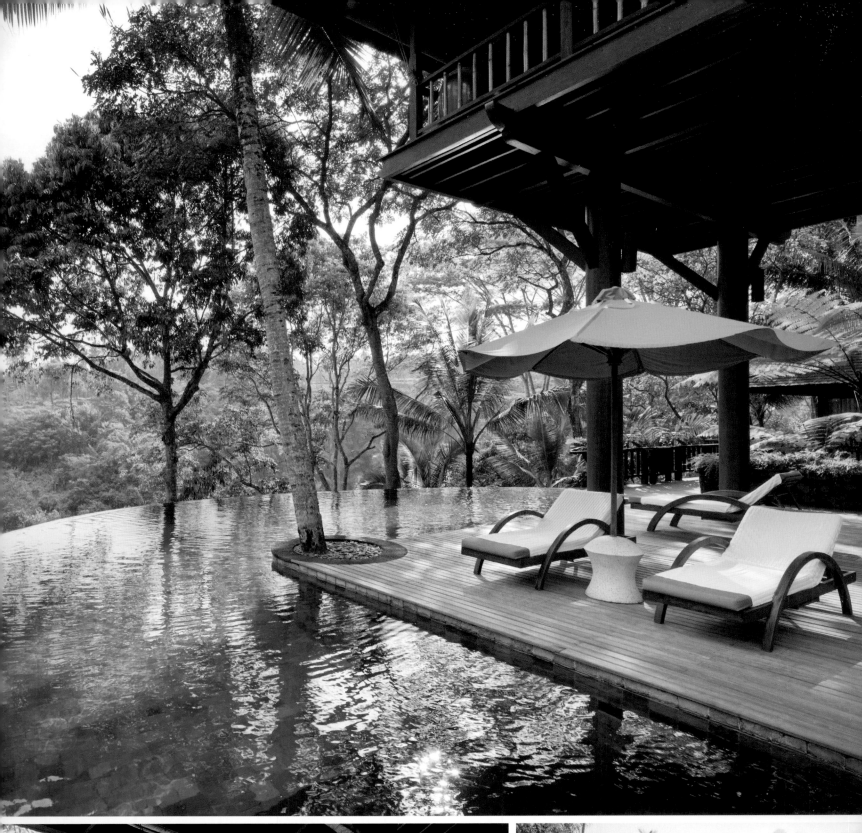

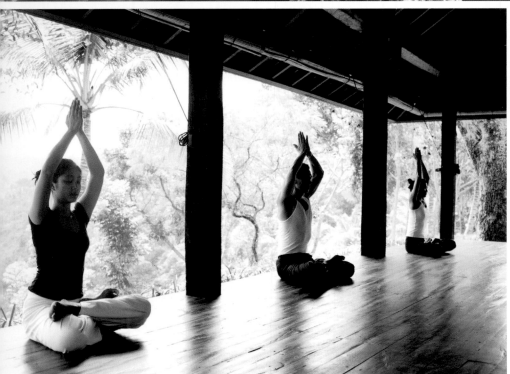

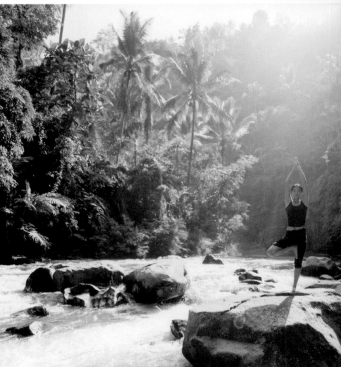

from above to below, from left to right: Wanakasa pool, sitting yoga, yoga on Ayung

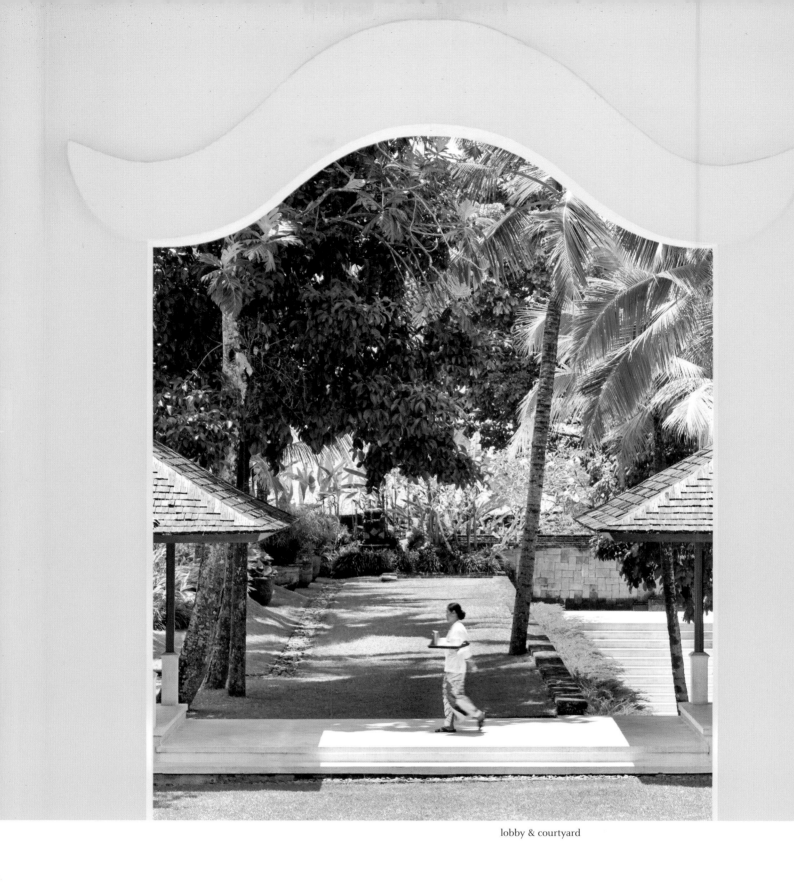

lobby & courtyard

COMO Shambhala Estate

Bali, Indonesia

Architect:
Cheong Yew Kuan
Location: Banjar Begawan,
Desa Melinggih Kelod,
Payangan, Ubud, Gianyar,
Bali 80571 Indonesia
Year of completion: 2005
Type of retreat: spiritual
retreat

COMO Shambhala Estate is a residential health retreat with luxury mansion-style accommodations near Ubud, Bali. This "Retreat for Change" is a place to relax and improve wellbeing. State-of-the-art wellness facilities include a Vitality pool, private treatment areas beside the river Ayung, a climbing wall, gym, Pilates studio and yoga pavilion. The Estate's Resident Experts, who all support the 360-degree approach to wellness, include a Yoga Master, Ayurvedic doctor and guides for outdoor activities, with nutritional menus by COMO Shambhala Cuisine. The range of suites and mansions, perched above the Balinese jungle, is suitable for single guests, couples, or small groups.

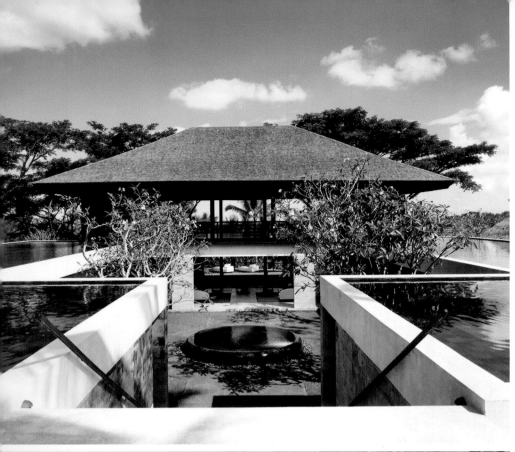

from above to below, from left to right: Ojas building, water garden, suite, villa with pool

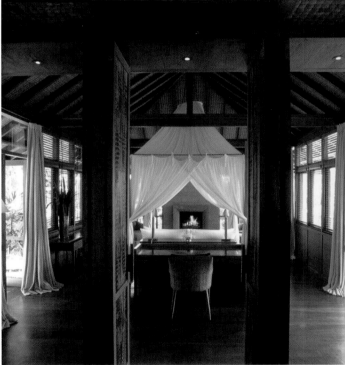

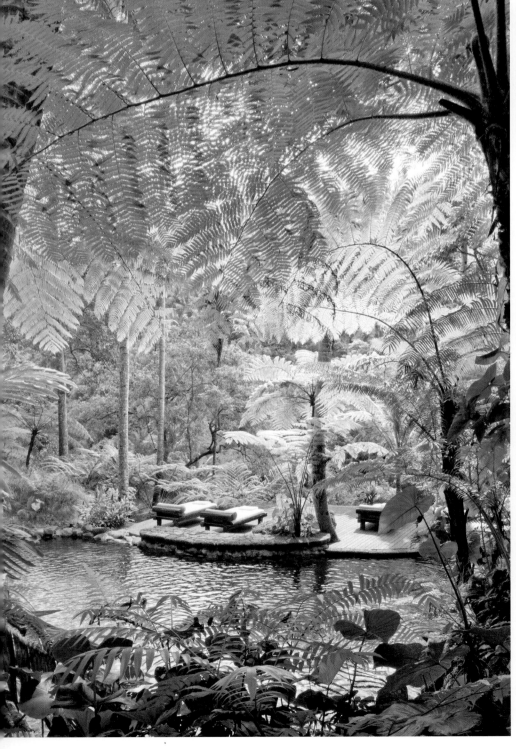

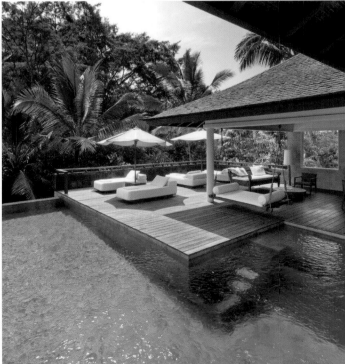

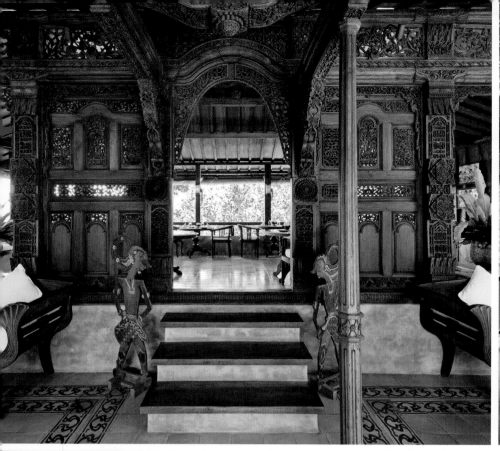

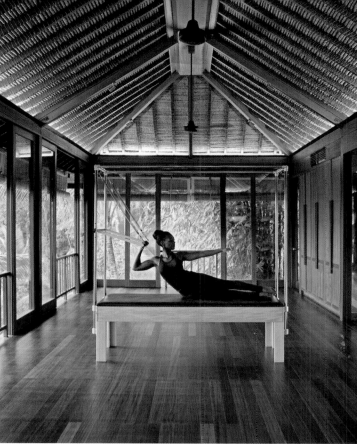

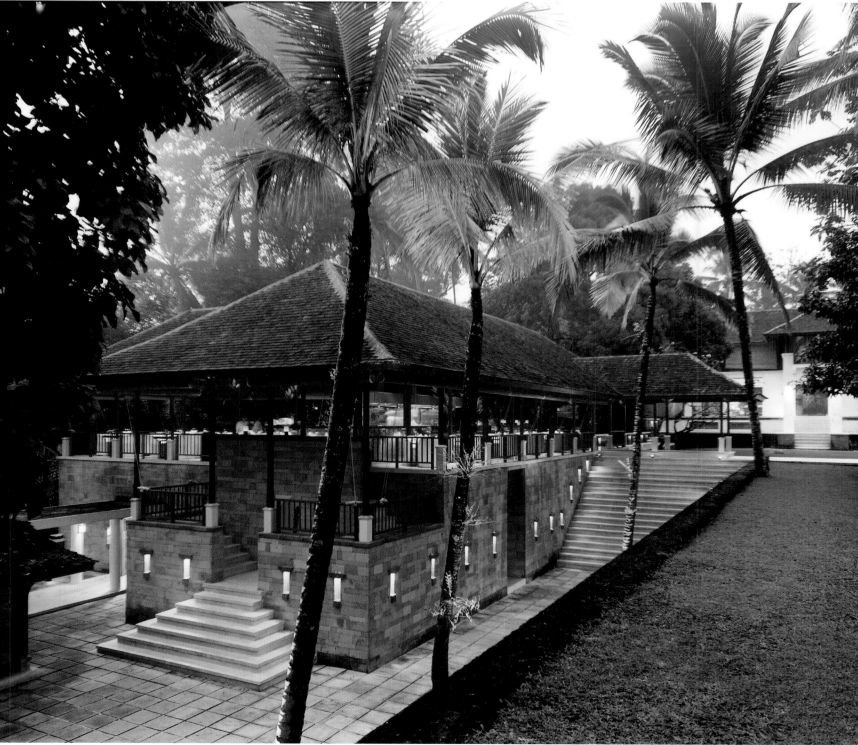

from left to right, from above to below: Kudus house, Pilates
studio, restaurant

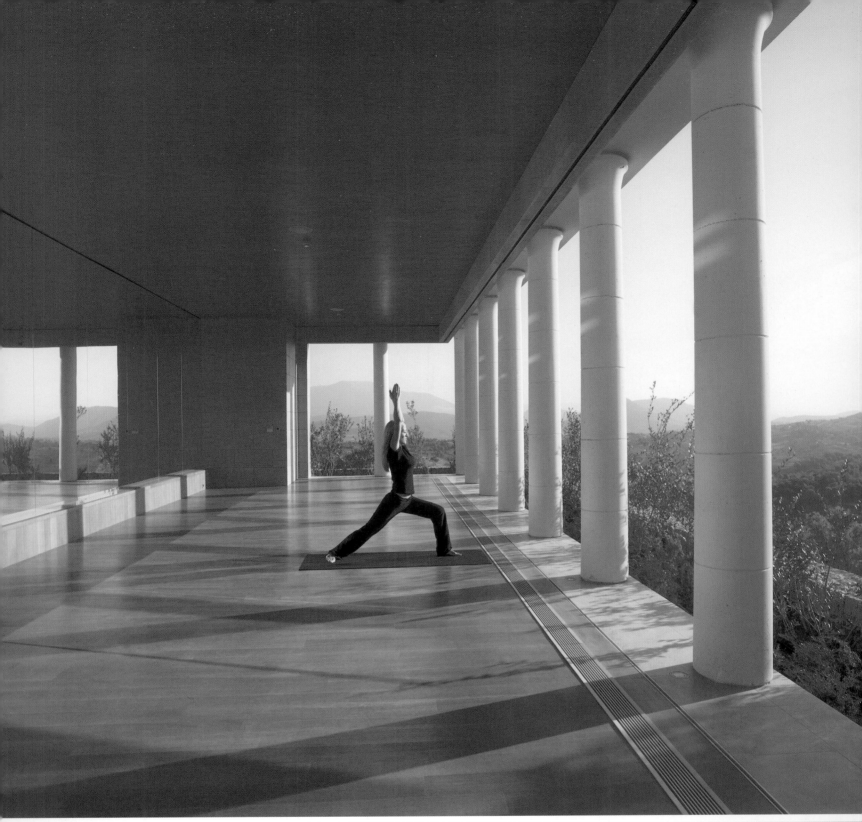

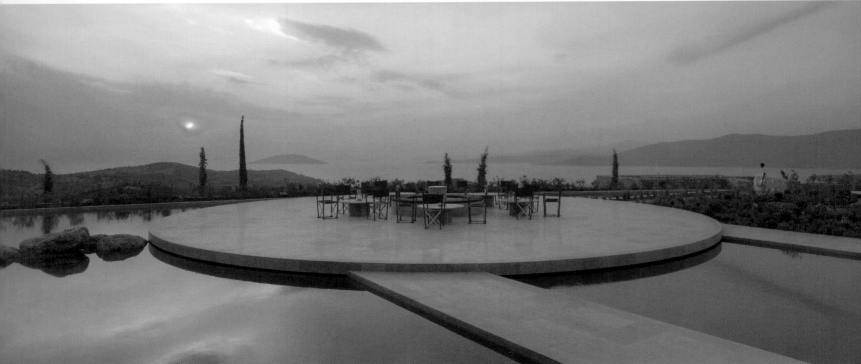

from above to below: yoga pavilion, central terrace

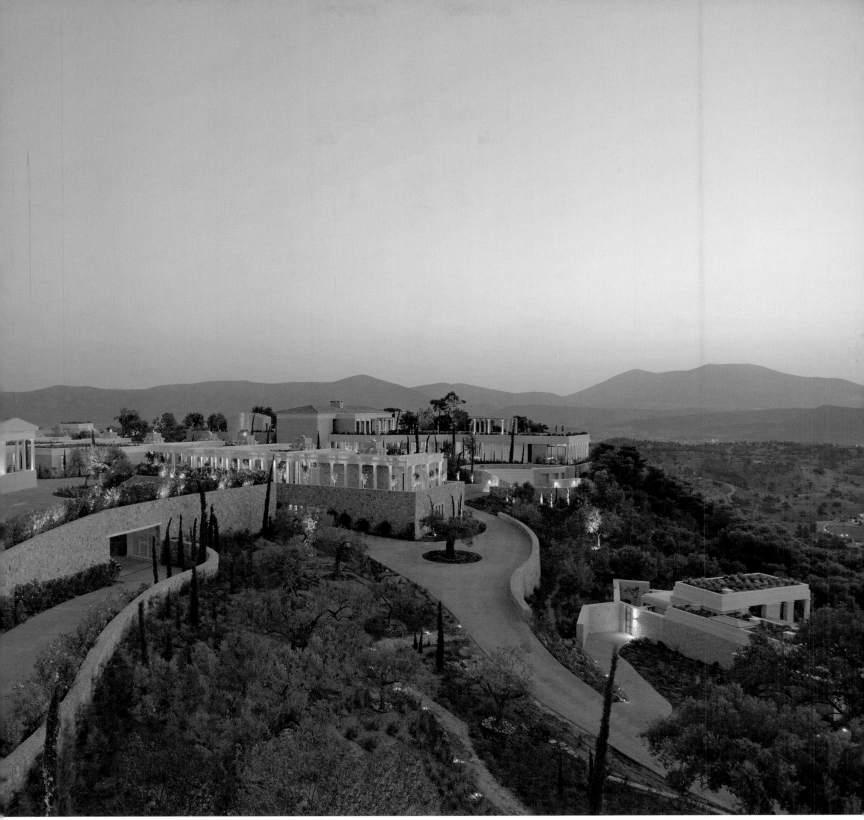

entrance area and pavilions

Amanzoe

Argolida, Greece

Architect: Ed Tuttle
Location: Aigos Panteleimonas, Kranidi, Argolida, 21300 Greece
Year of completion: 2012
Type of retreat: resort

Surrounded by undulating olive groves, Amanzoe features 38 pavilions and overlooks the turquoise waters of the Aegean Sea. The design is strongly influenced by classical Greek architecture, yet is contemporary in attitude and construction techniques. The reception areas overlook a reflection pool, beyond which the library, boutique and gallery are set amongst terraces, courtyards and gardens.

The dining pavilions and lounges include the restaurant, pool restaurant, fireplace and living room with its central bar. The landscape allows for several secondary areas such as the Aman Spa, the main swimming pool with terrace, a gym, Pilates studio and yoga pavilion and a small amphitheater. The beach club is just a 10-minute drive from the resort.

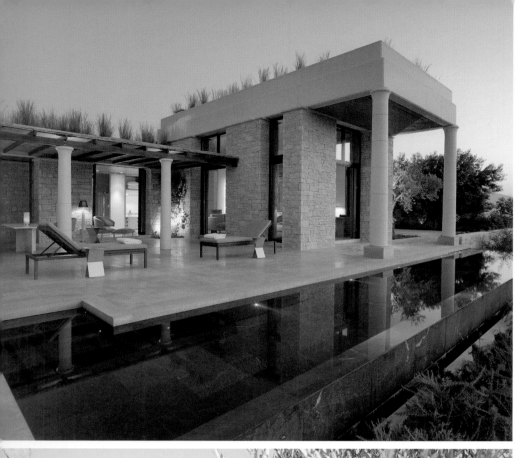

from above to below, from left to right: pool pavilion, bedroom, swimming pool

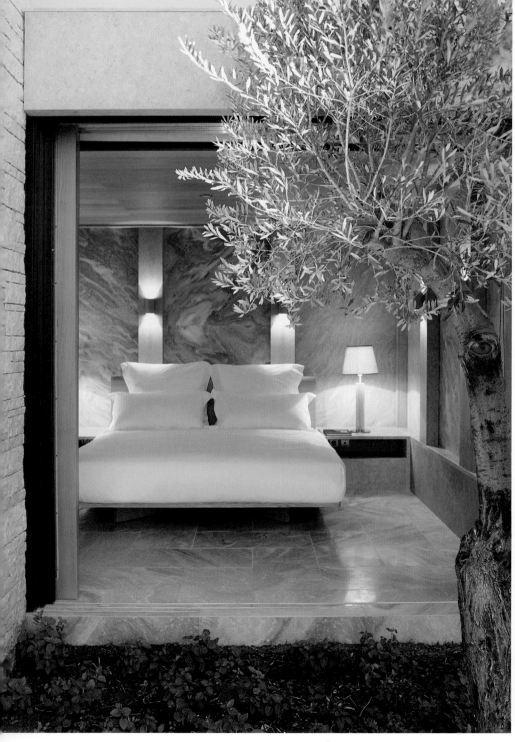

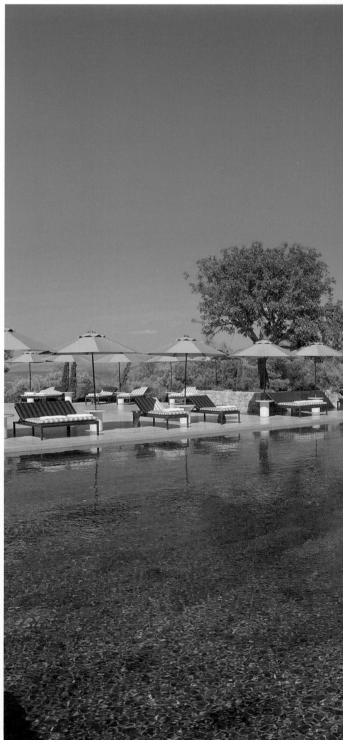

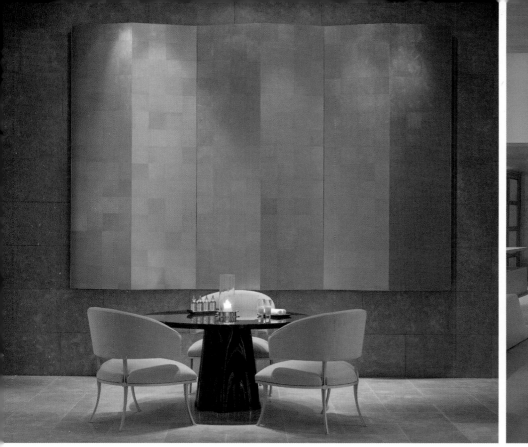

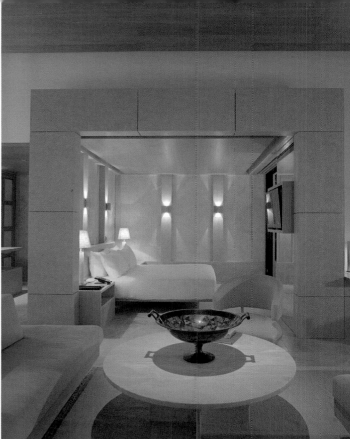

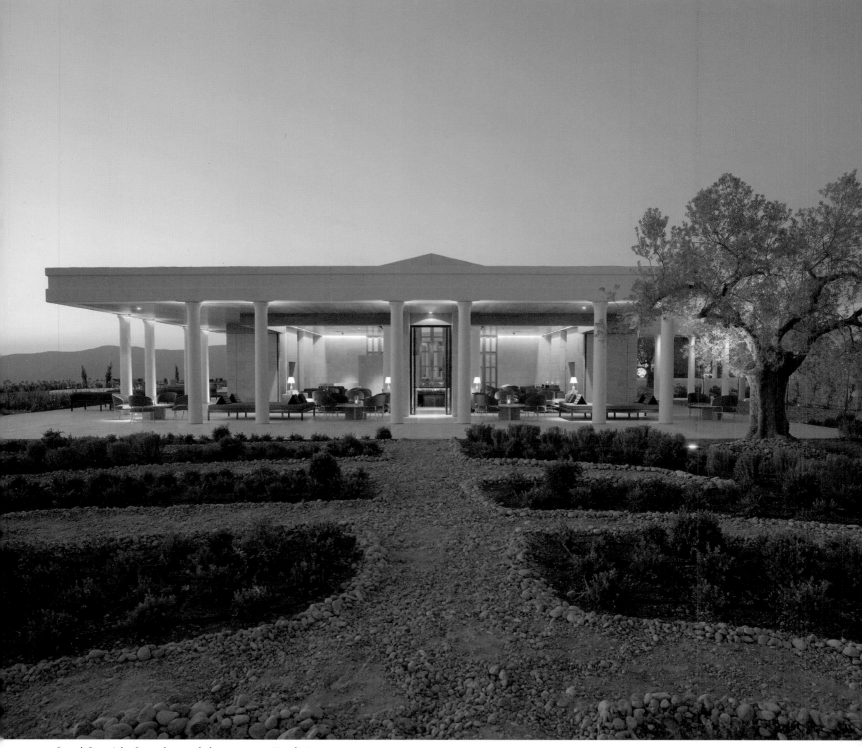

from left to right, from above to below: spa reception, living
room, exterior view

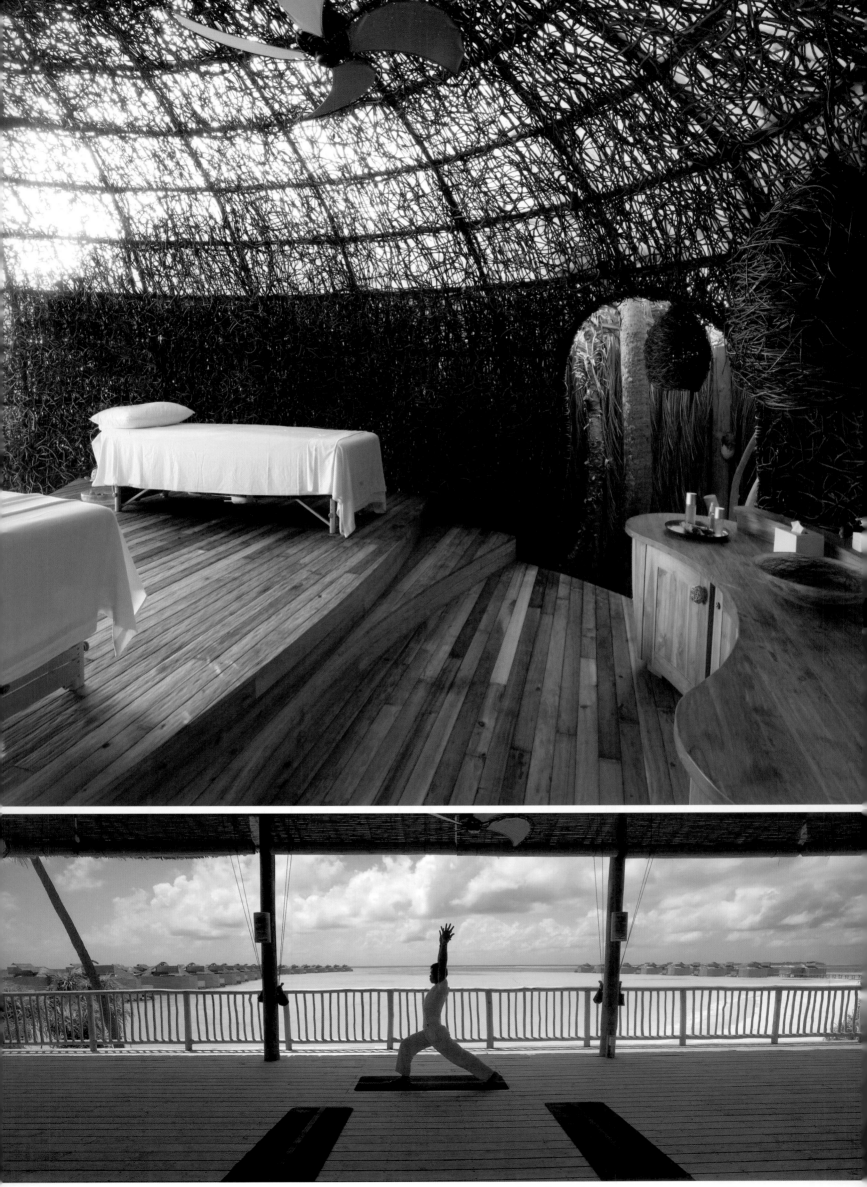

from above to below: treatment room, yoga pavilion

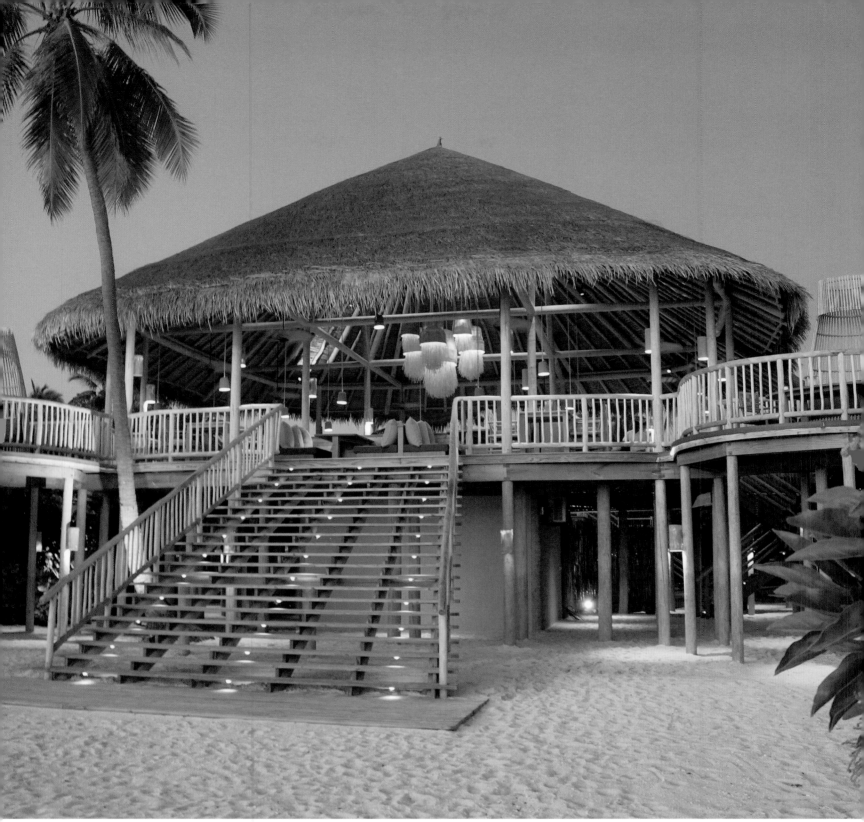

exterior view

Six Senses Laamu

Laamu Atoll, Maldives

Architect:
Habita Architects
Location: Olhuveli Island,
Laamu Atoll,
Maldives
Year of completion: 2011
Type of retreat: hotel,
resort and spa

Six Senses Laamu is the only resort in the Laamu Atoll, deep in the Indian Ocean, surrounded by a beautiful coral house reef. Although most of the mansions and facilities are built overwater, beach mansions and on-land dining are options. All mansions offer a sense of privacy and seclusion, with an amazing view of the ocean and Maldivian nature. Six Senses Laamu offers a wide range of dining options, with cuisines from around the world, an ice cream parlor, an overwater wine cellar and a signature chill bar. Many activities, excursions and options are available for everyone to enjoy, both over and under water, in addition to the Six Senses Spa.

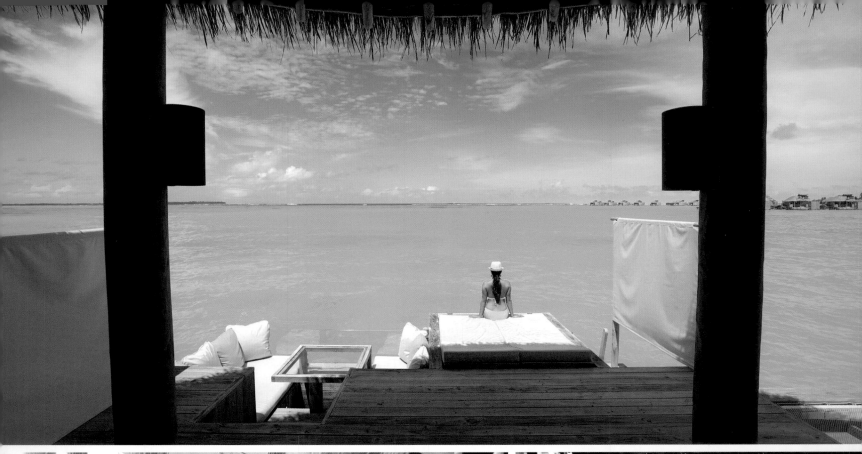

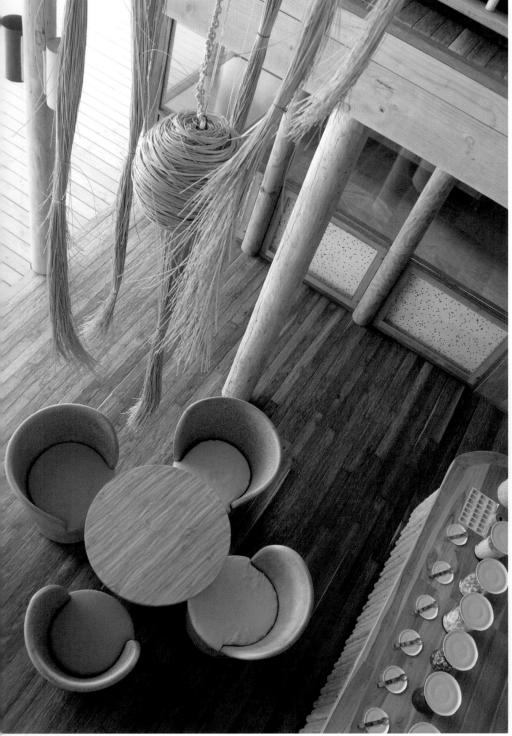

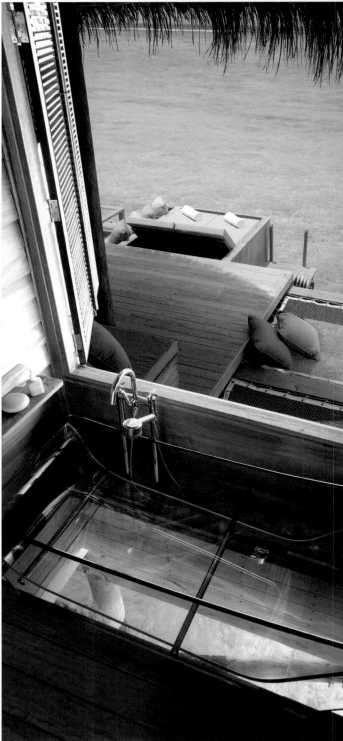

from above to below, from left to right: villa on the sea, interior view, bath

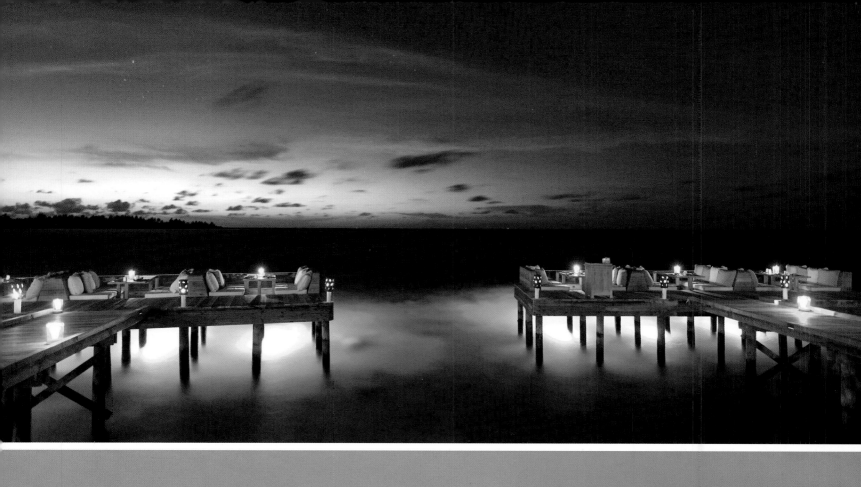

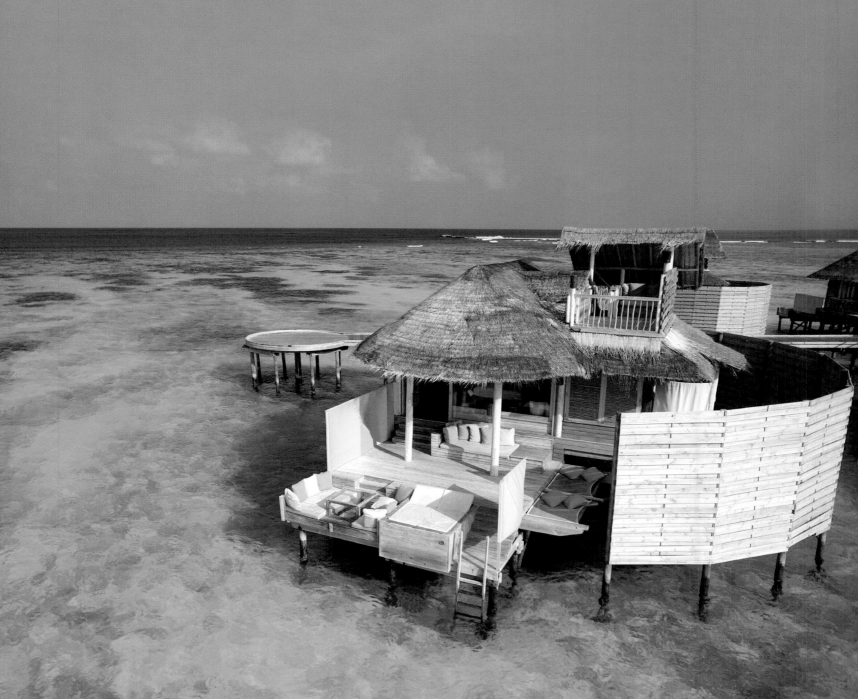

from above to below: Atoll at night, Atoll at day

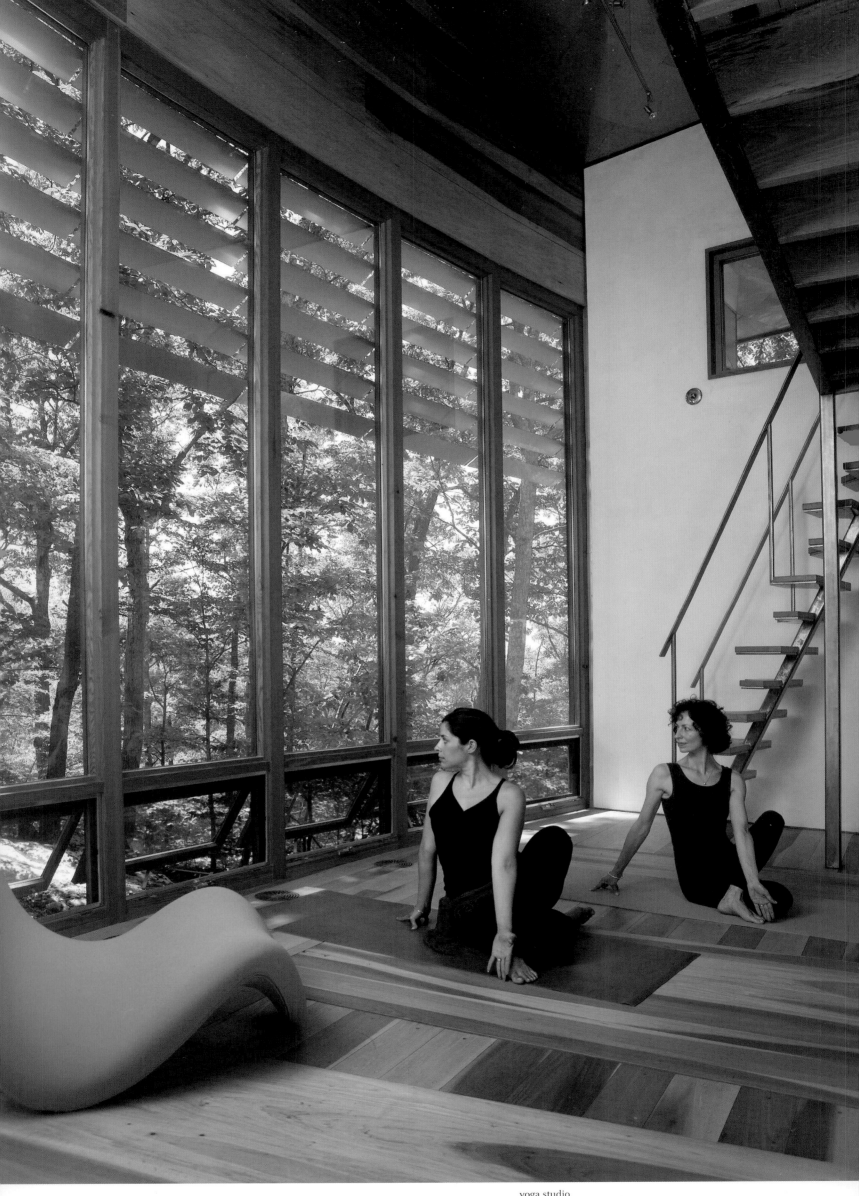

yoga studio

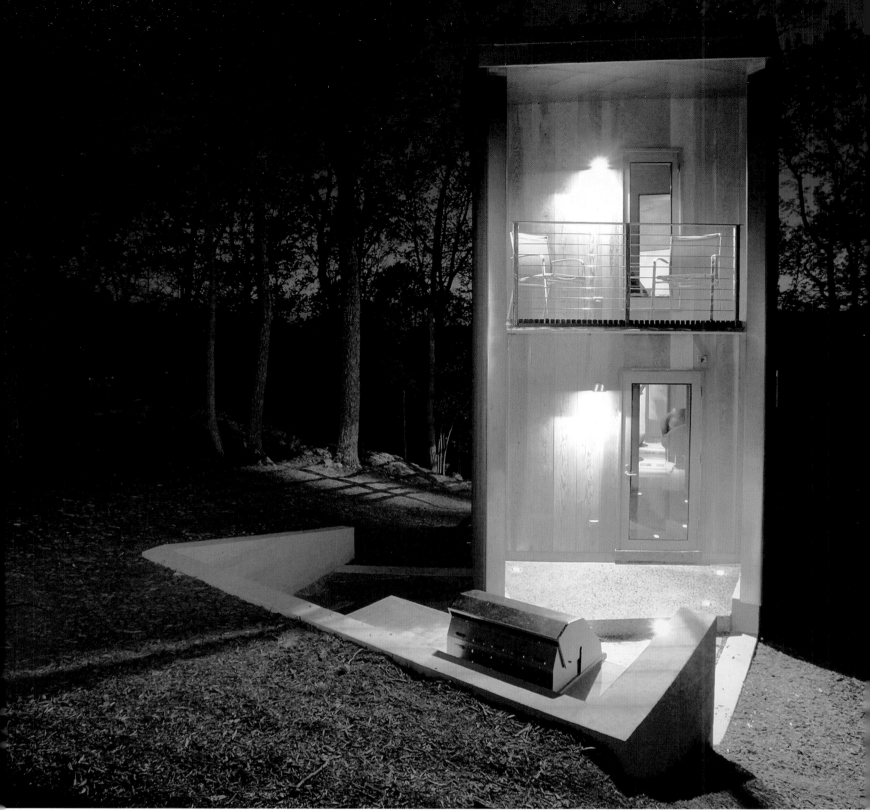

exterior view

Yoga Studio
Virginia, USA

Architect: Carter + Burton Architecture P.L.C
Location: Clarke County, Virginia, USA
Year of completion: 2007
Area: 55,742 sqm
Type of retreat: yoga studio

The owners, both practicing Buddhists and avid modernists, were interested in creating a weekend retreat from Washington, DC in the Shenandoah Valley. The natural setting with distant vistas and nearby rock outcropping maintain an atmosphere of enjoyment for the meditation. An organic shape takes in as much southern light as possible while still being compact. The morphology of the curved interior space inside transports all who visit it. This outbuilding fits with the site while maintaining a modern purity of form and space rarely seen in a rural setting. A high bermed entrance to the east and the western end with a deck on the side with the view feels like a tree house. The details, materials, furniture and nature provide the only artistic expression, freeing the space of metaphysical distractions.

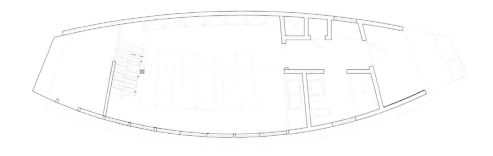

from above to below, from left to right: floor plan, back deck,
living area

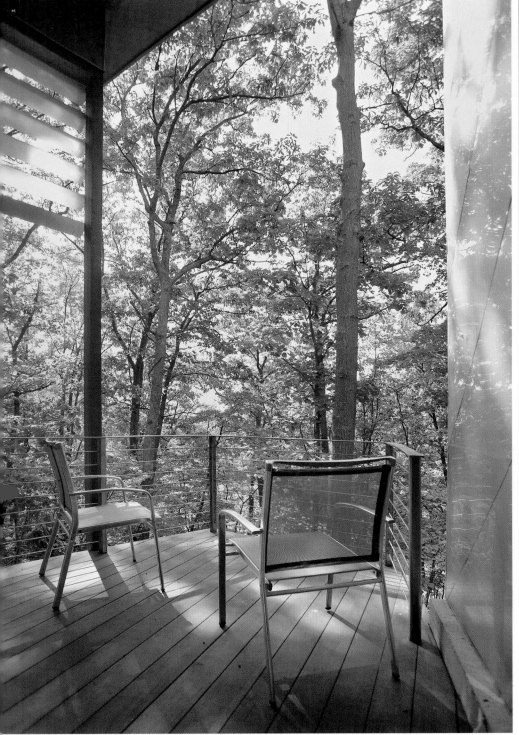

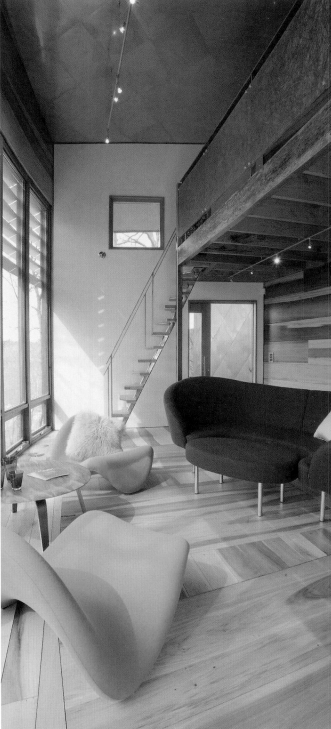

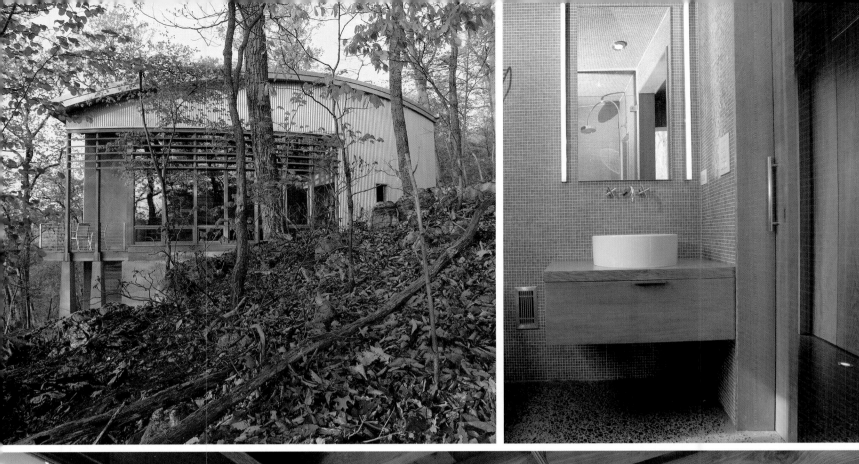

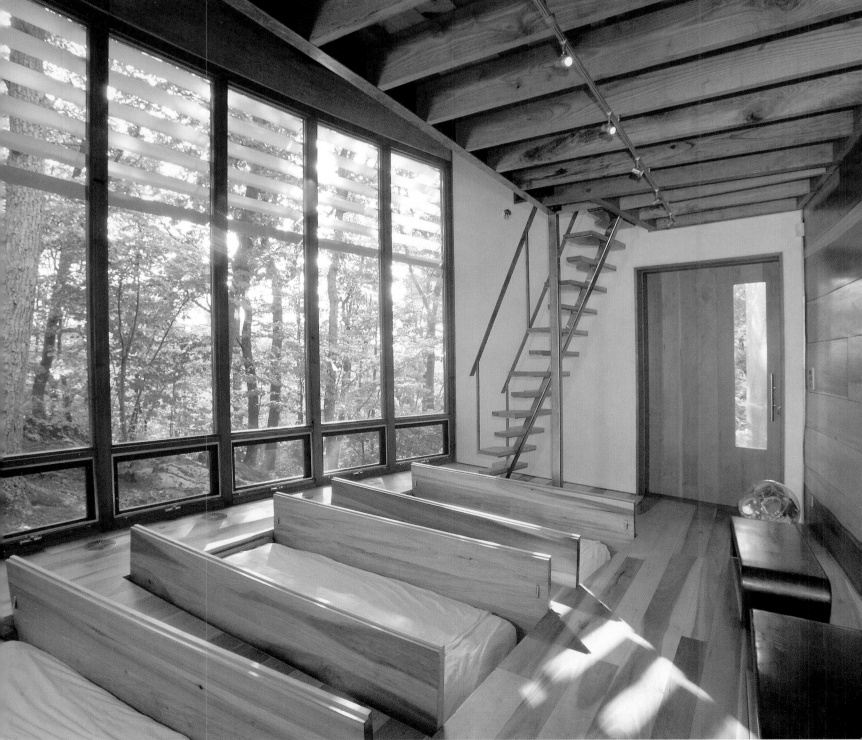

from left to right, from above to below: southern exposure,
bathroom, under loft

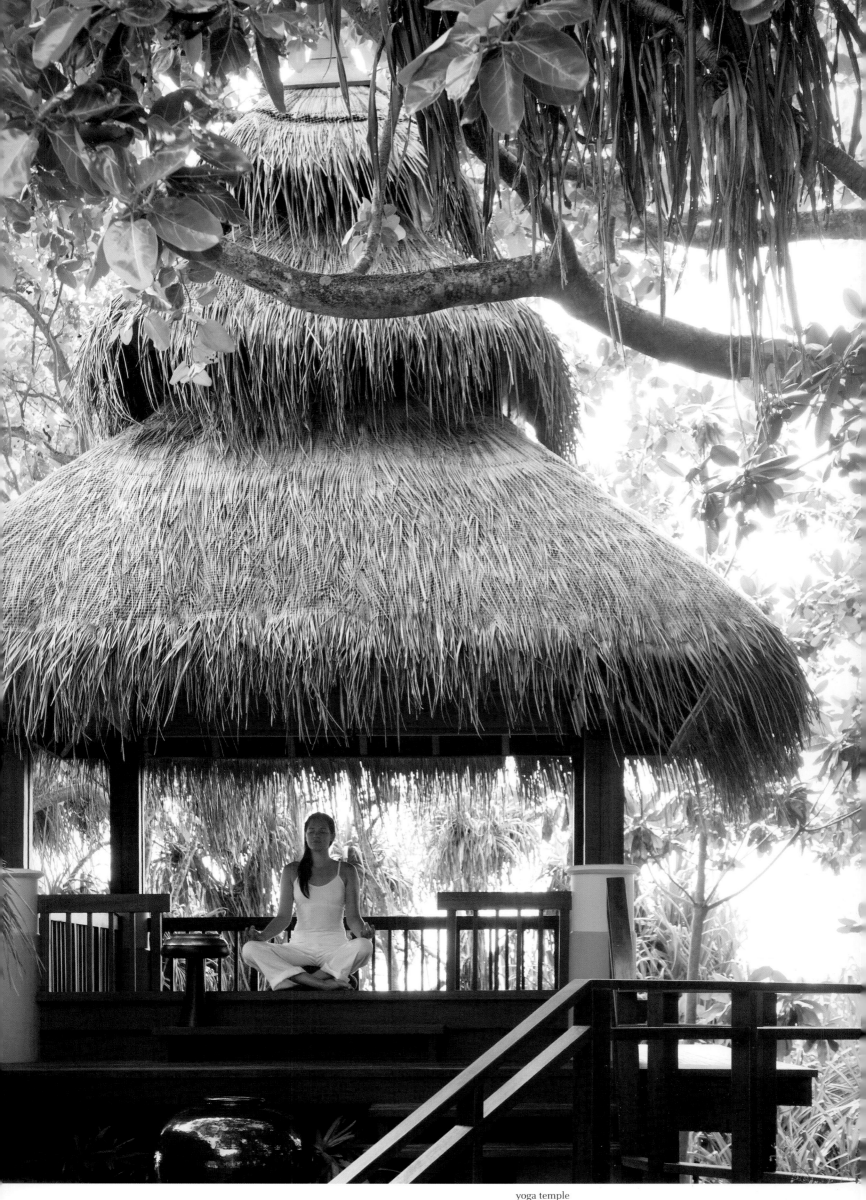

yoga temple

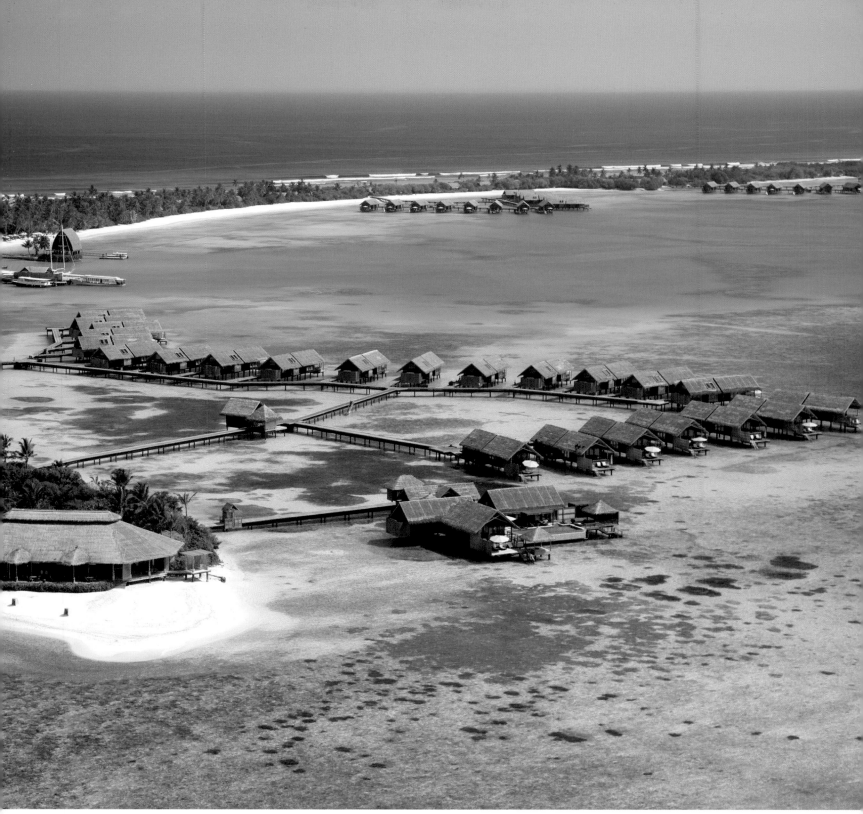

aerial view

Shangri-La's Villingili Resort & Spa

Villingili Island, Maldives

Architect: Wimberly Allison Tong & Goo
Designer: Lim Teo+Wilkes Design Works
Location: Villingili Island, Addu Atoll, Maldives
Year of completion: 2009
Area: 120,000 sqm
Type of retreat: resort & spa

The Shangri-La Villingili Resort & Spa opened in 2009 as the first luxury resort in the Addu Atoll south of the equator. There is enough island romantic for the guests to enjoy on the two kilometer long white sand beach. But Villingili has much more to offer: 29 acres of lush vegetation with 17,000 palms and old Banyan fig trees, three natural lagoons and a nature trail over and under water.

The spa is located on the highest point of the island. With eleven spa mansions, the spa complex is the largest in the Maldive Islands. The program is based on philosophies and rituals from China and the Himalayas. It employs element analysis, which is based on the Chinese Yin and Yang philosophy. Guests become familiarized with their personal elements – metal, water, wood, fire or earth.

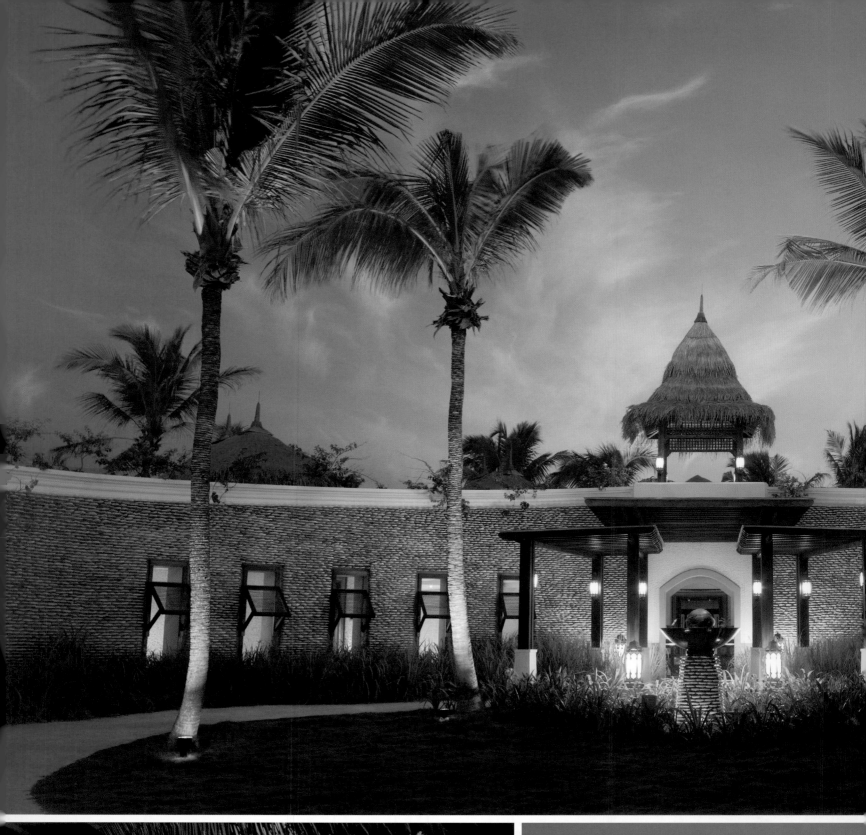

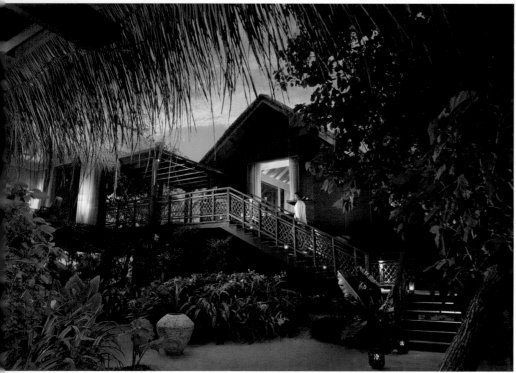

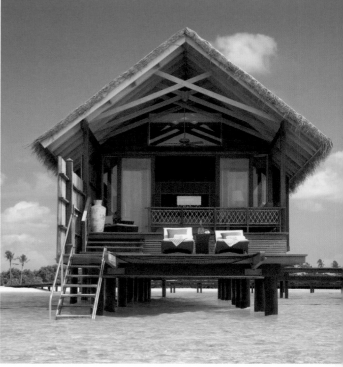

from above to below, from left to right: entrance area, exterior
view, waterside view

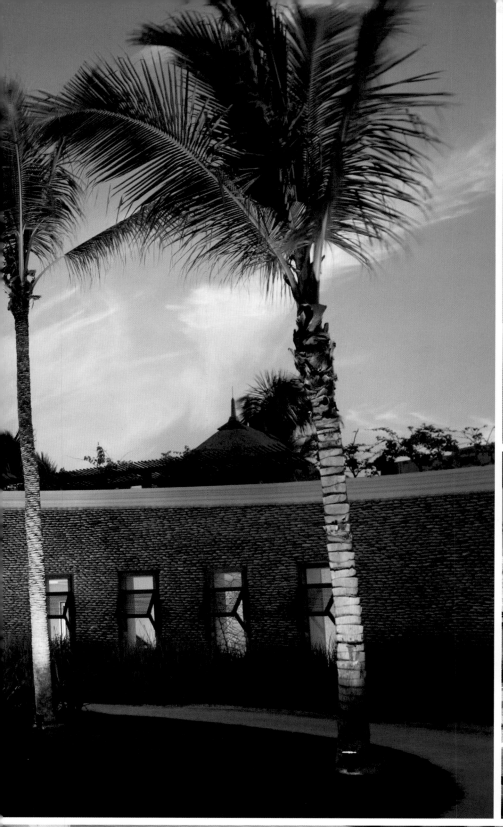
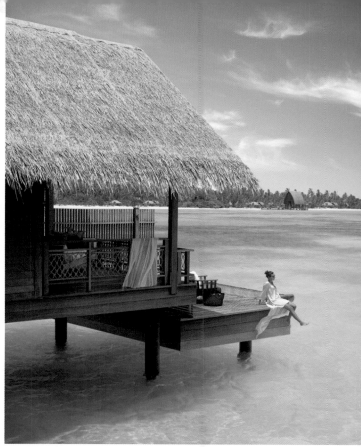
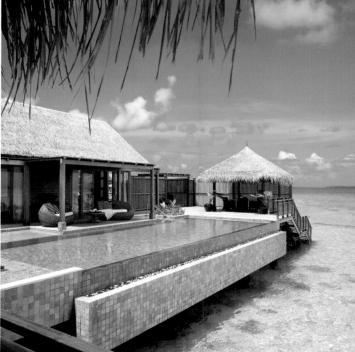
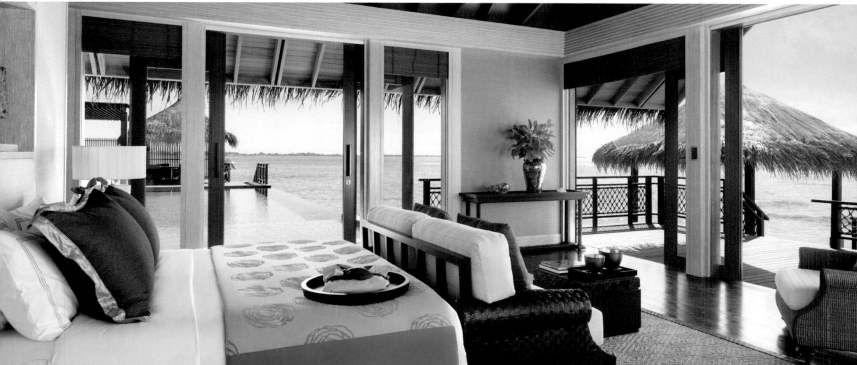

from above to below, from left to right: villa with ocean view,
outdoor pool, bedroom

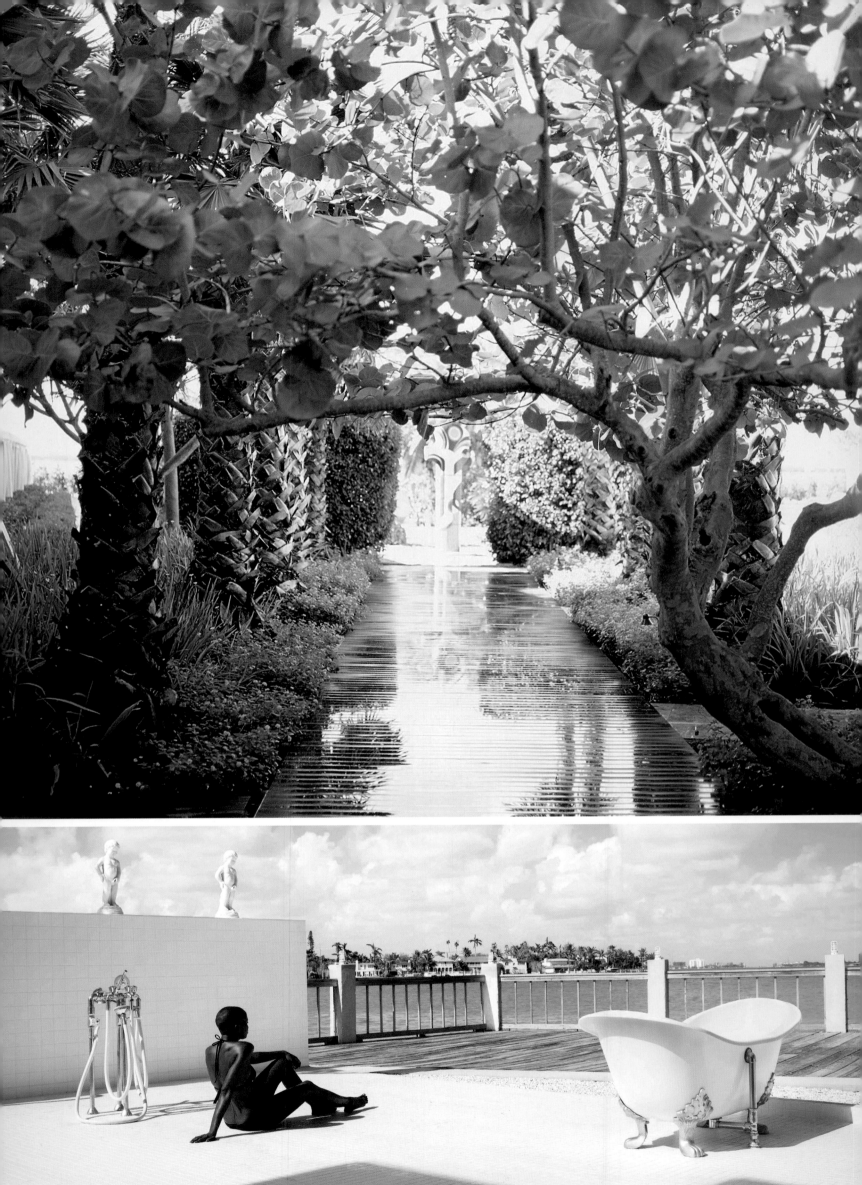

from above to below: garden view, mud baths

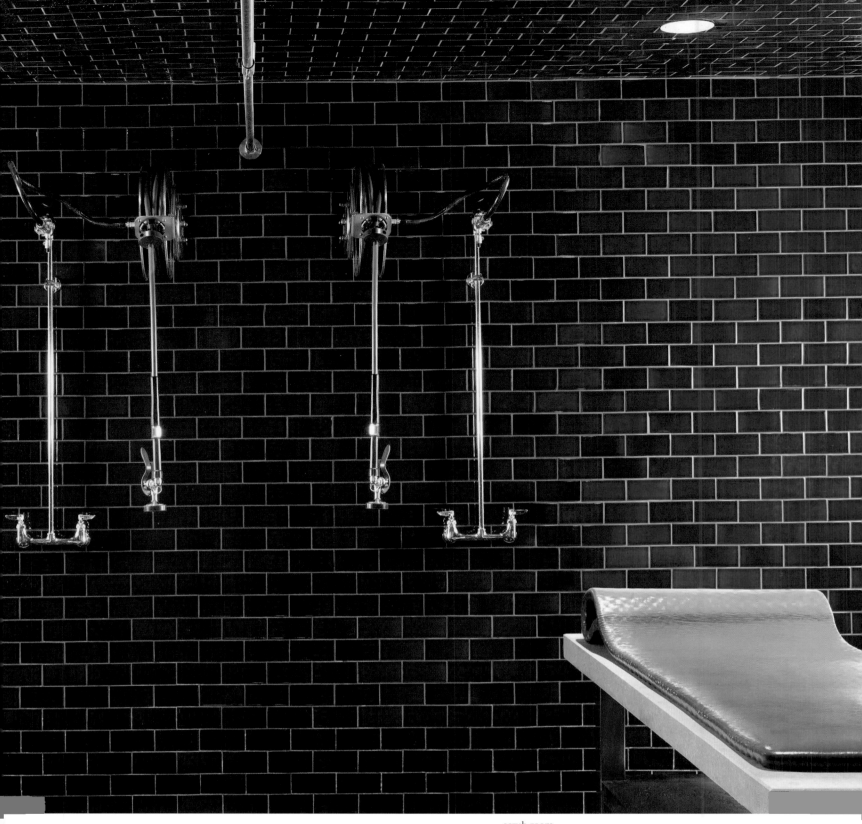

scrub room

The Standard

Miami, USA

Architect: Allison Spear Architect
Location: 40 Island Avenue, Miami Beach, FL 33139, USA
Year of completion: 2011
Type of retreat: spa & yoga

Hotel's architectural history: The Standard aka Lido Spa was originally designed in 1953 by Norman M. Giller & Associates and consisted only of the two hotel guest room wings. Norman Giller was one of the originators of the motel concept in Florida. The front building – often incorrectly attributed to Morris Lapidus – was actually designed by A. Herbert Mathes Architect. The front building was constructed in 1960. In 2005 the property was renovated into the Standard by Allison Spear Architect.

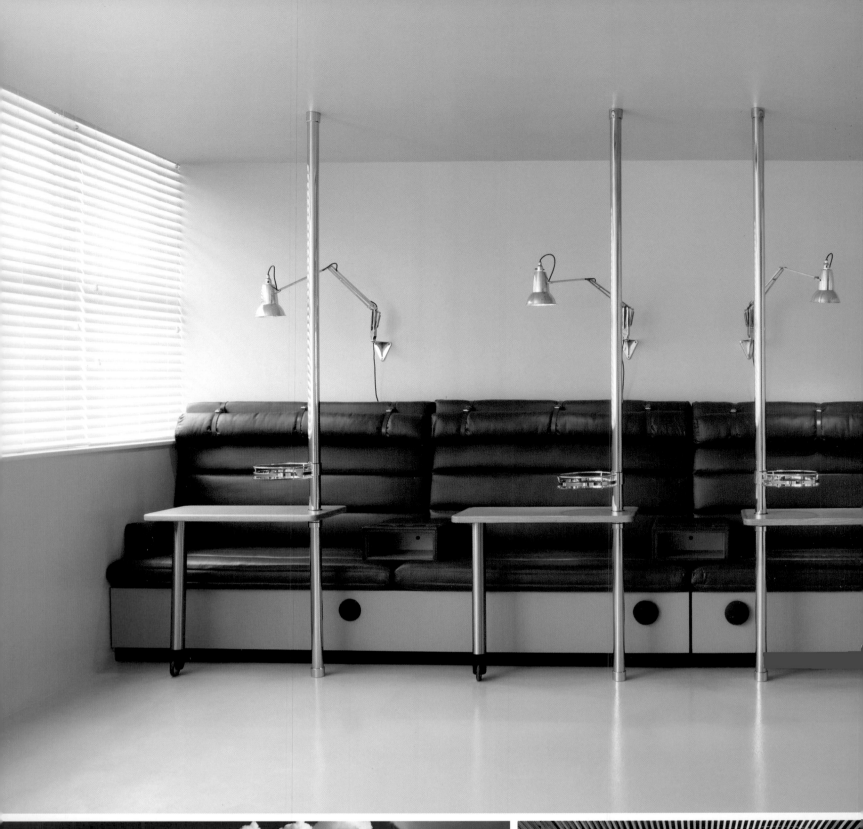

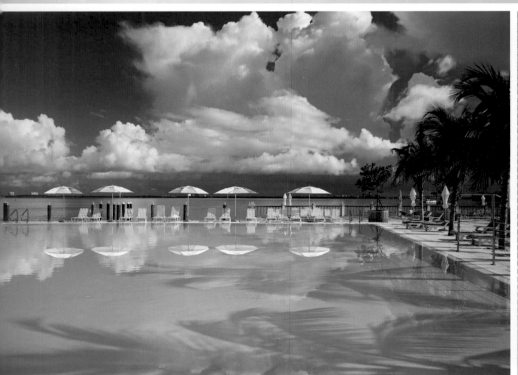

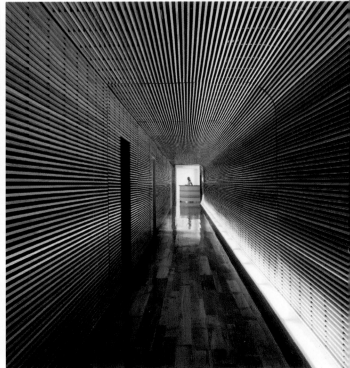

from above to below, from left to right: pedicure room,
exterior pool, hallway

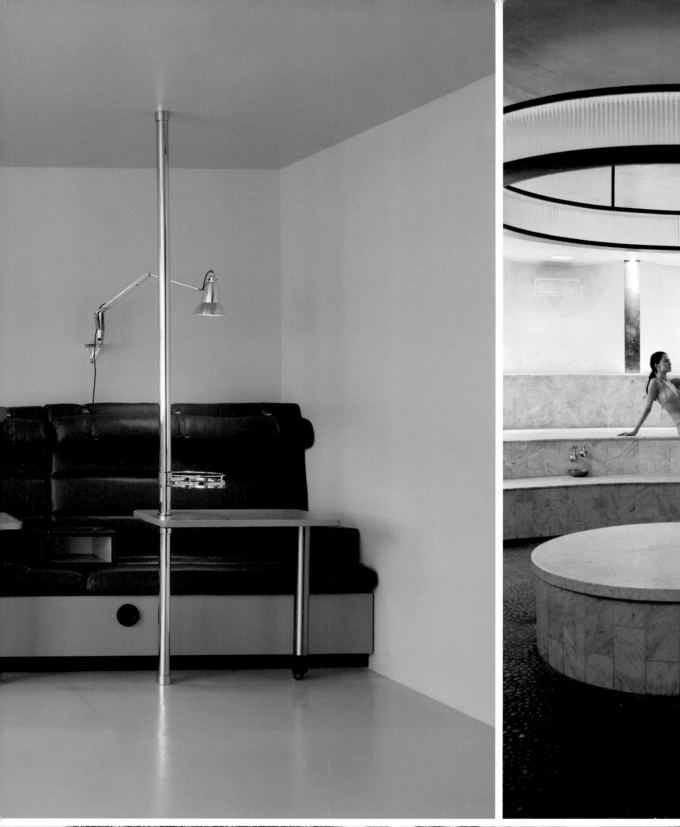

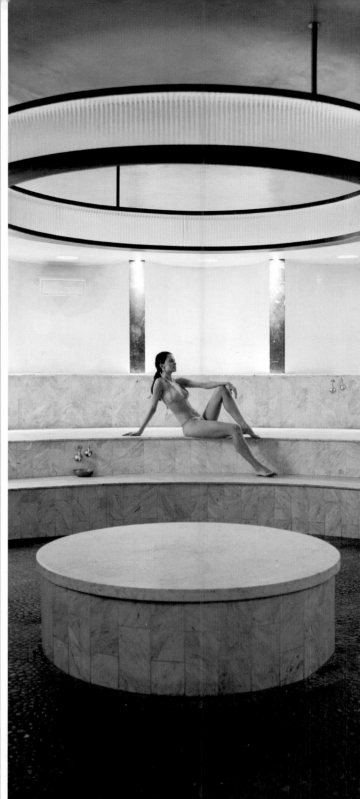

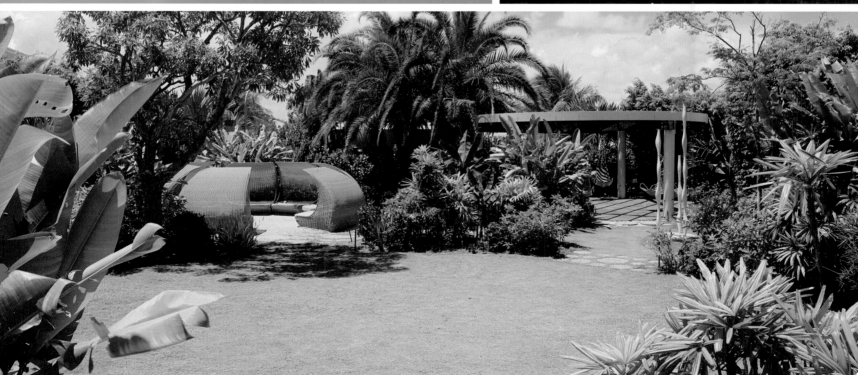

from above to below: hammam, garden

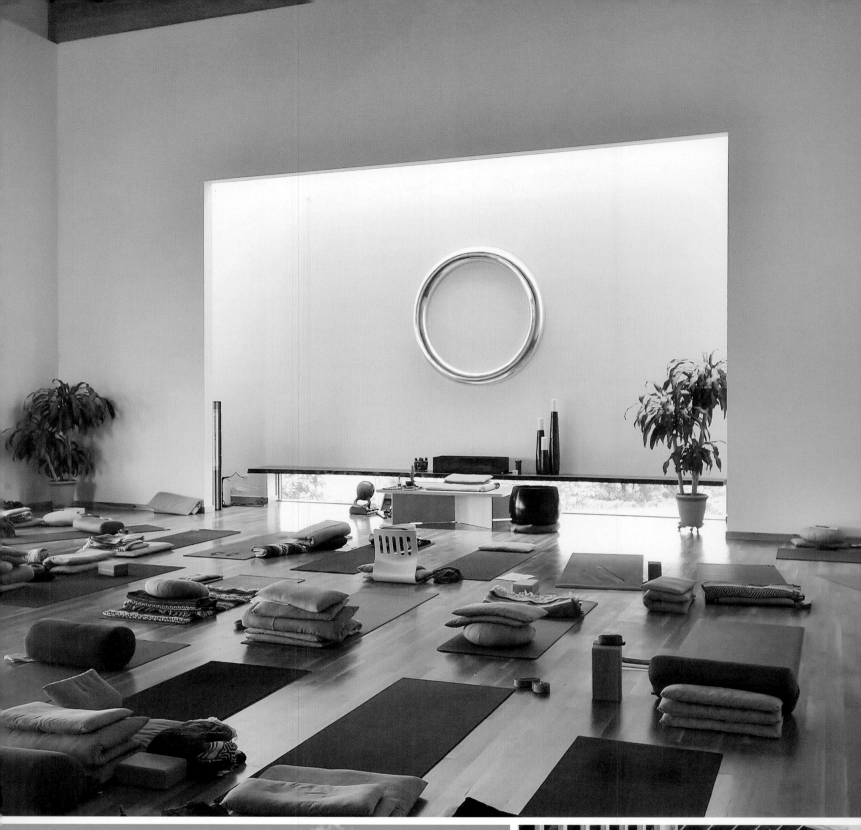

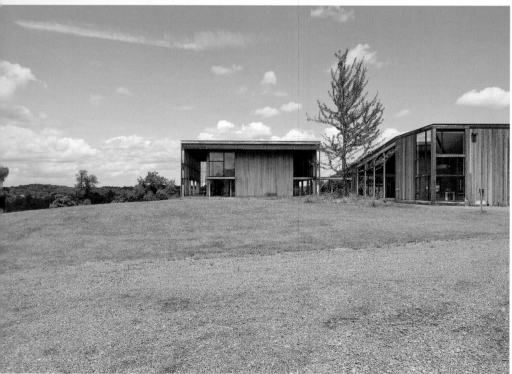

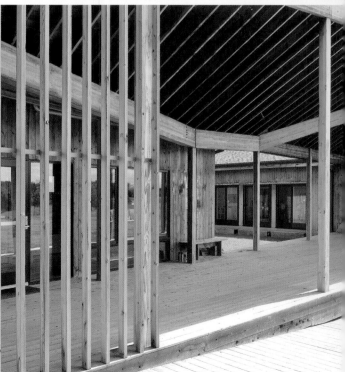

from above to below, from left to right: meditation space,
meditation hall and administration, entrance area

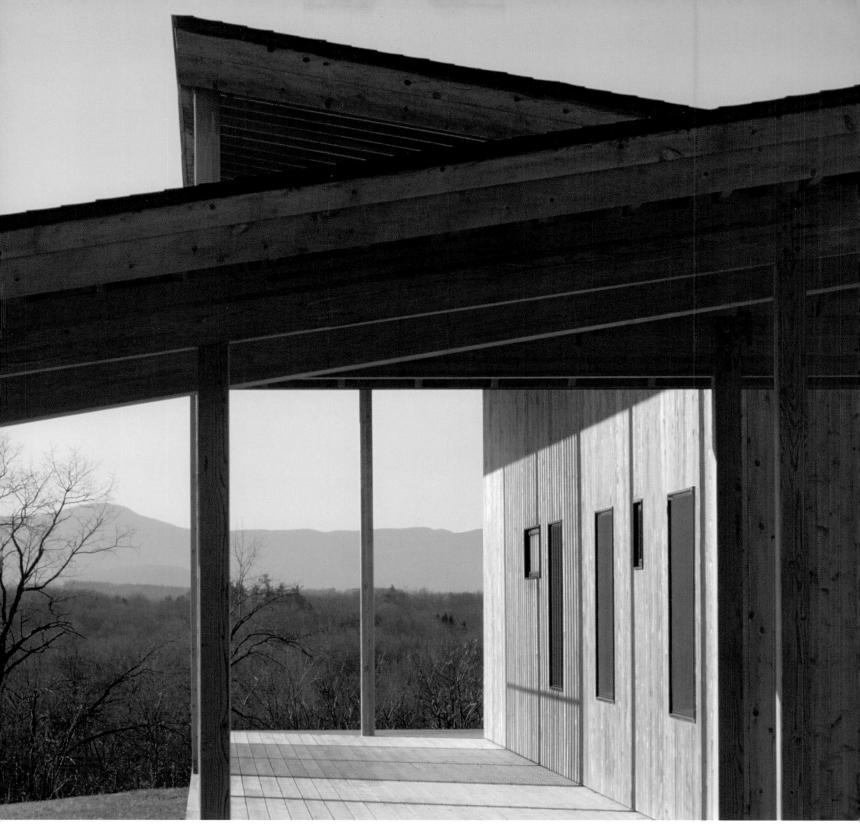

permanent residence porch

Won Dharma Center

Claverack, USA

Architect: Hanrahan Meyers Architects LLP
Location: 361 Route 23, Claverack, NY 12513, USA
Year of completion: 2012
Area: 3,000 sqm
Type of retreat: spiritual, Buddhist meditation retreat

The Won Dharma Center is a 3,000 square meter spiritual and recreational retreat in Claverack, New York for the Won Buddhists, a Korean organization that emphasizes balance in daily life and a relationship to nature. The center is designed for a zero-carbon footprint and is located within a 500-acre property on a gently sloping hill with views to the west of the Hudson River valley and the Catskills. The symbol of the Won organization is an open circle, suggesting both a void without absence and infinite return. The buildings are organized around the dual concepts of the void and spiral.

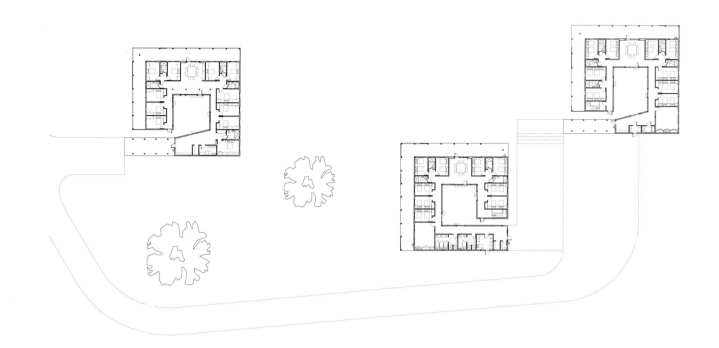

from above to below: site plan, guest residence porch

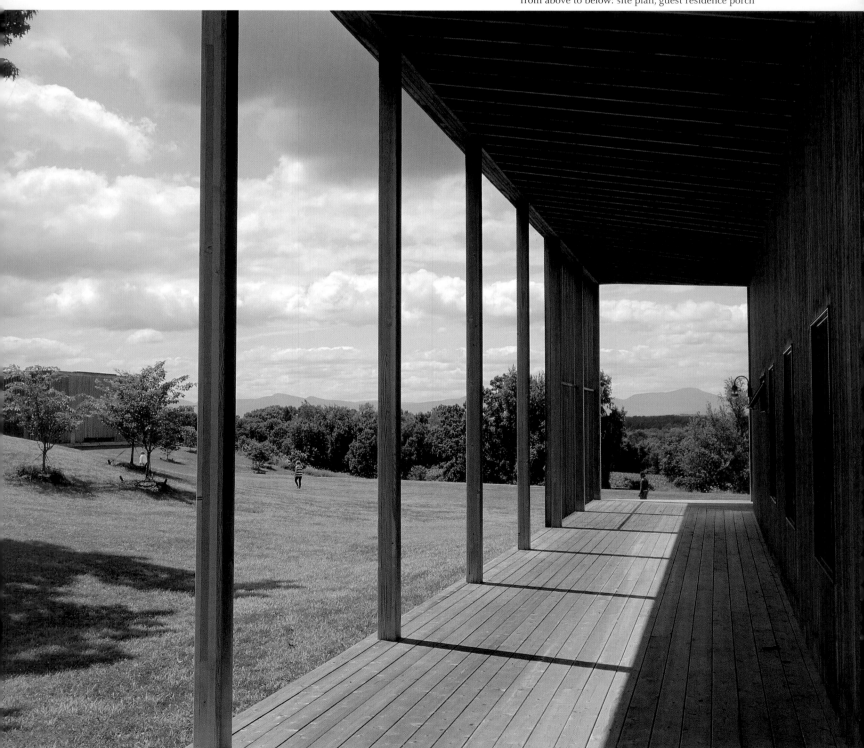

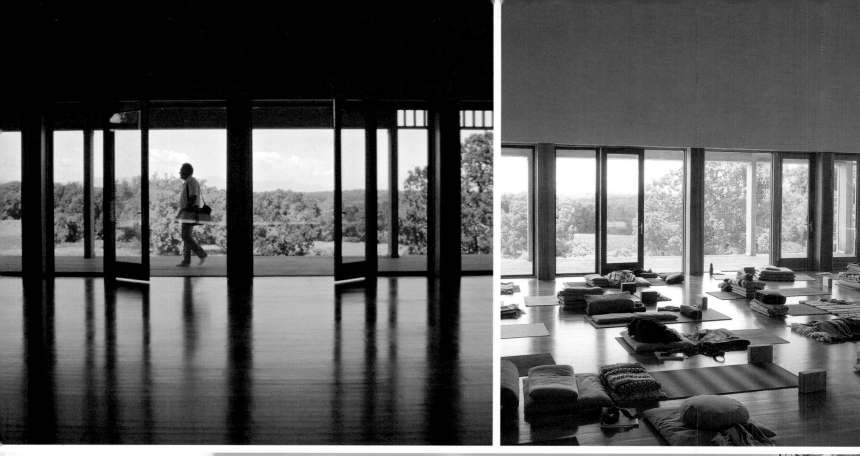

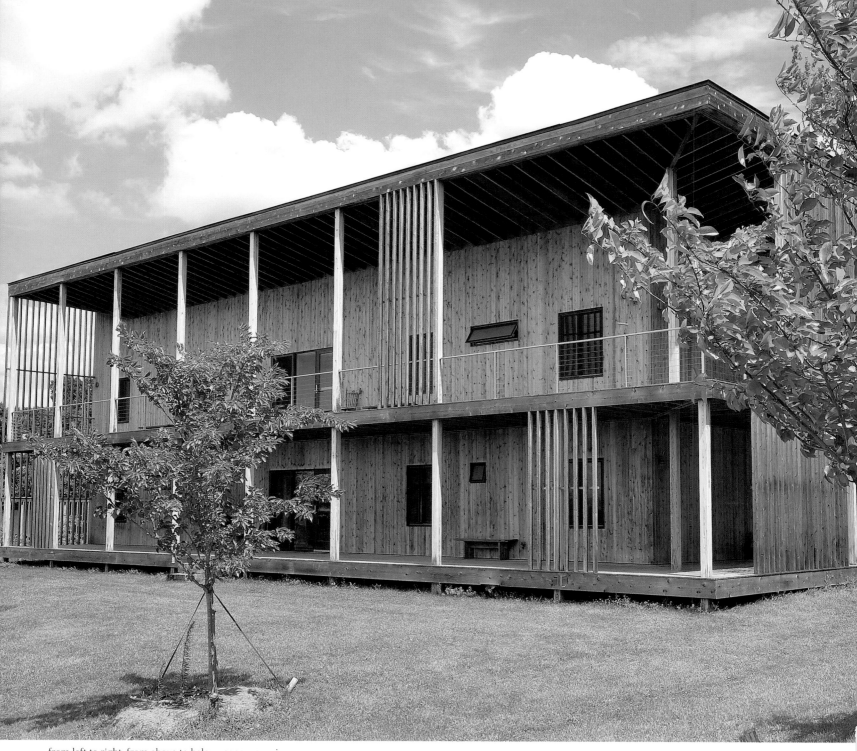

from left to right, from above to below: panorama view,
meditation room, permanent residence

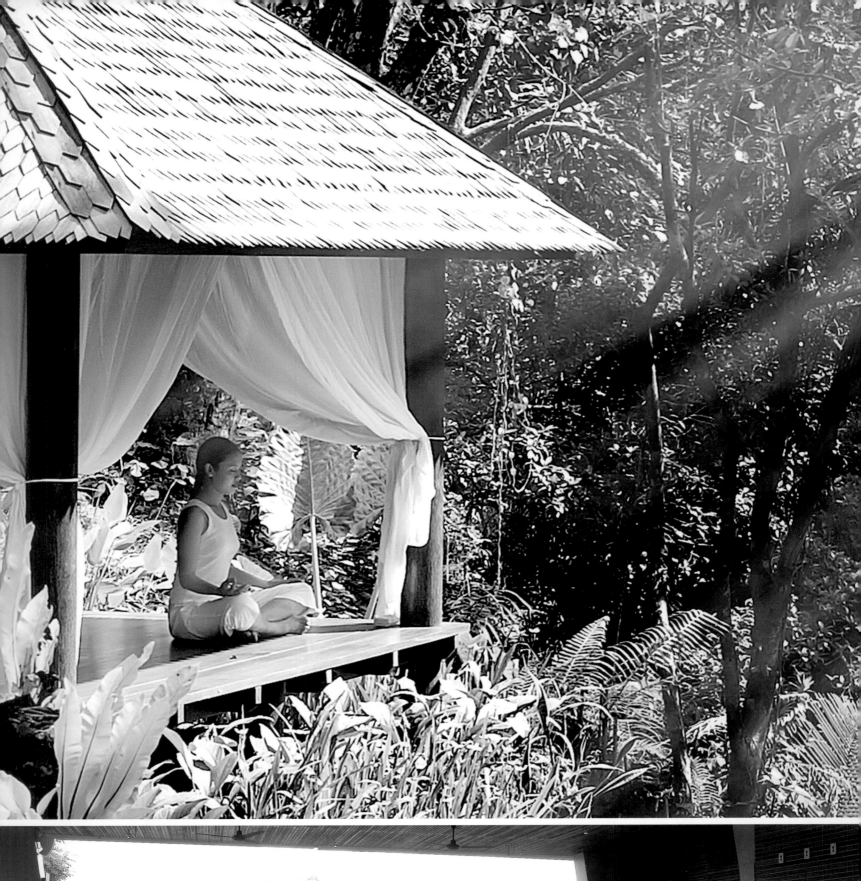

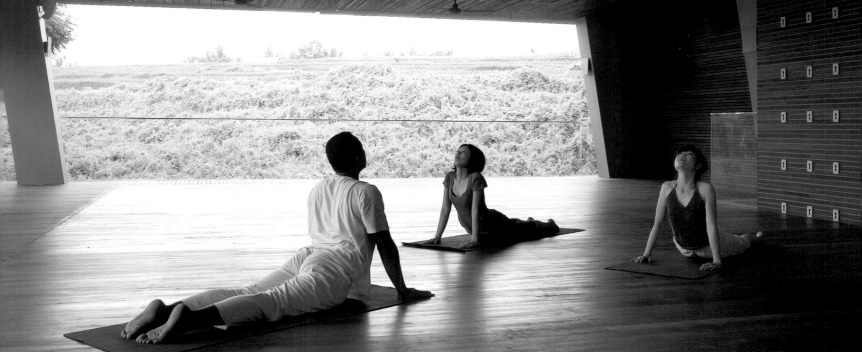

from above to below: meditation, yoga pavilion

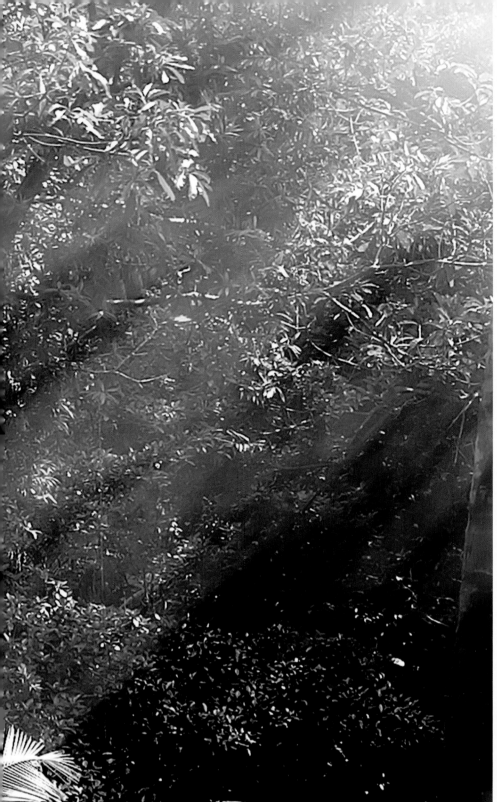
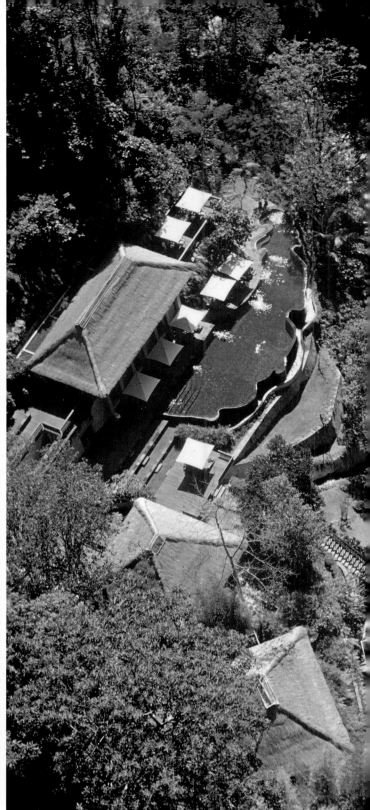

aerial view

Maya Ubud Resort & Spa

Ubud Bali, Indonesia

Architect: Budiman Hendropurnomo – Denton Corker Marshall
Location: Gunung Sari Street, Peliatan, Ubud Bali, Indonesia
Year of completion: 2001
Area: 120,000 sqm
Type of retreat: resort & spa

At Maya. a series of parallel lines are inspired by the Ancient Balinese tradition of orienting the villages along the Kaja – Kelod axis, linking Mount Agung in the center of the island to the surrounding seas. Some of these architectonic lines are represented by a series of four monumental stonewalls ranging from 125 to 155 meters length and up to 2.5 to 6 meters height. They look like what might be left after flooding had eroded the soil between them. In some locations, like the main axis linking the lobby and the spa, a strong line is carved into the landscape. Other lines are mere dots of old stone artifacts on a simple oval lawn or a series of stone benches. These monumental protrusions and depressions are the primary composition, where the rest of the architecture is attached.

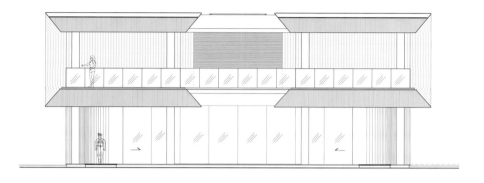

from above to below: front elevation, river view

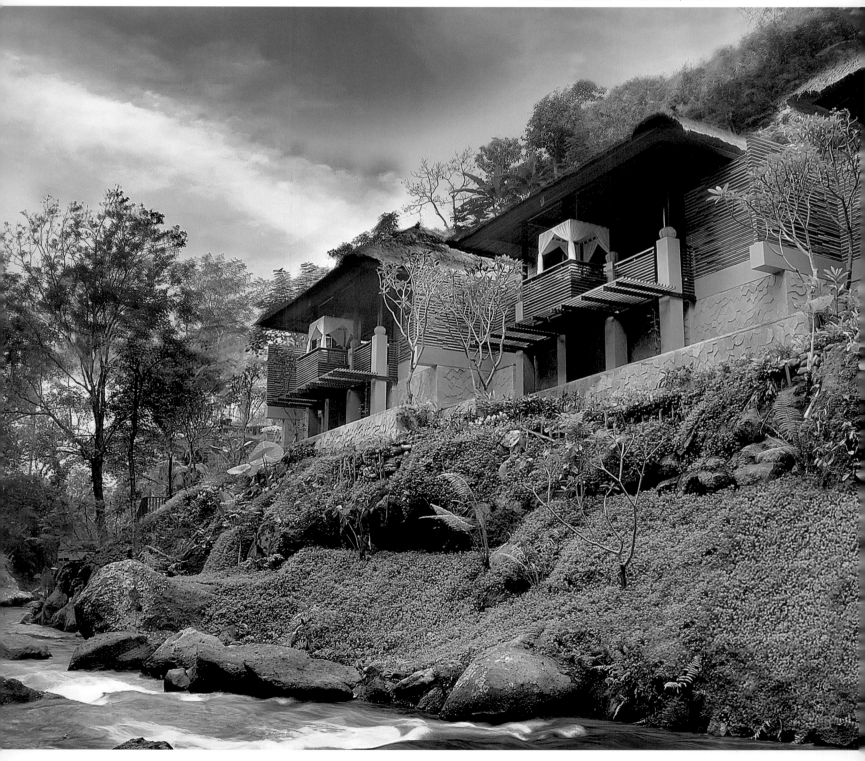

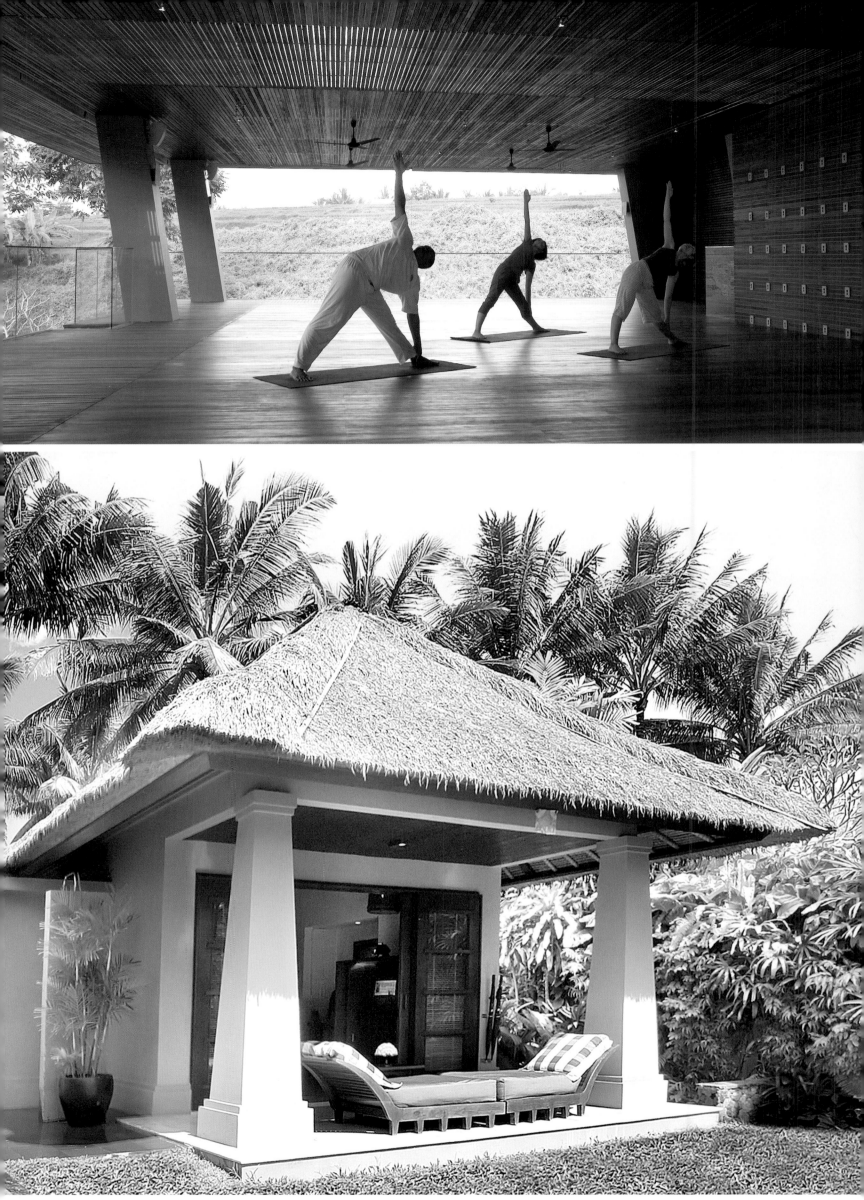

from above to below: yoga pavilion, pool villa

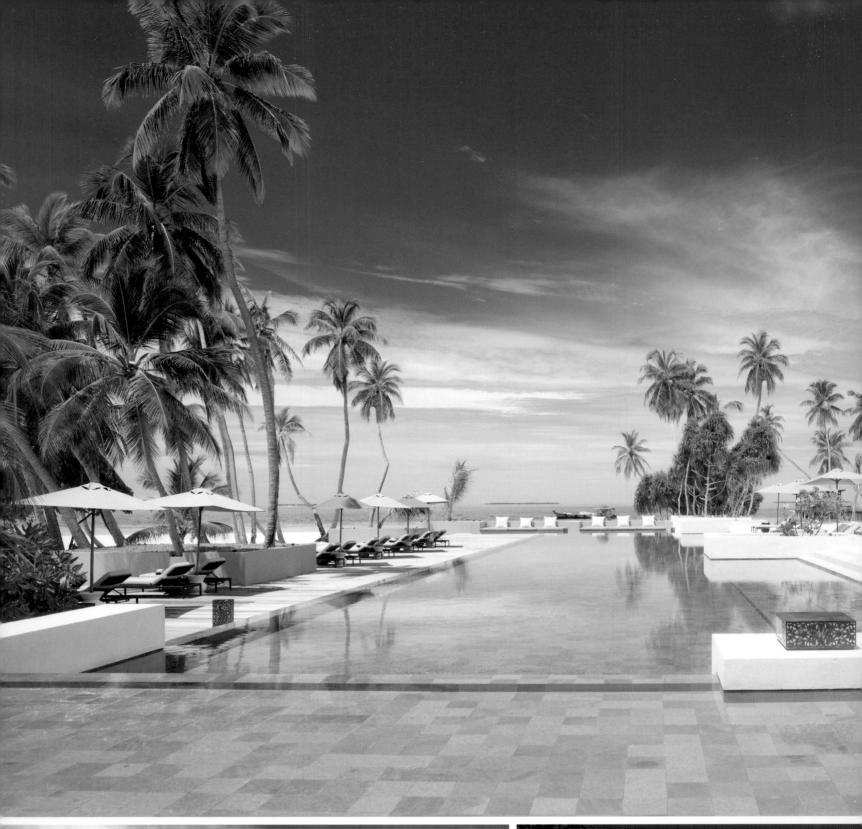

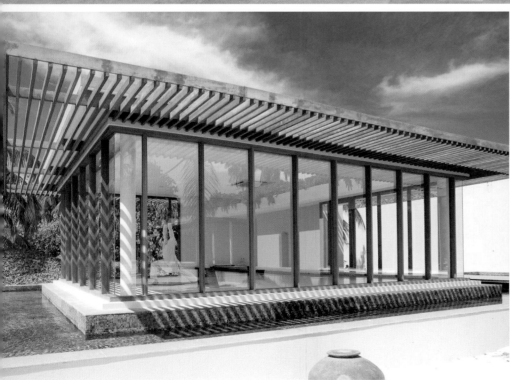

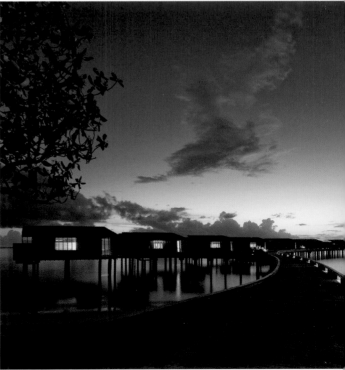

from above to below, from left to right: pool area, yoga pavilion, water villas

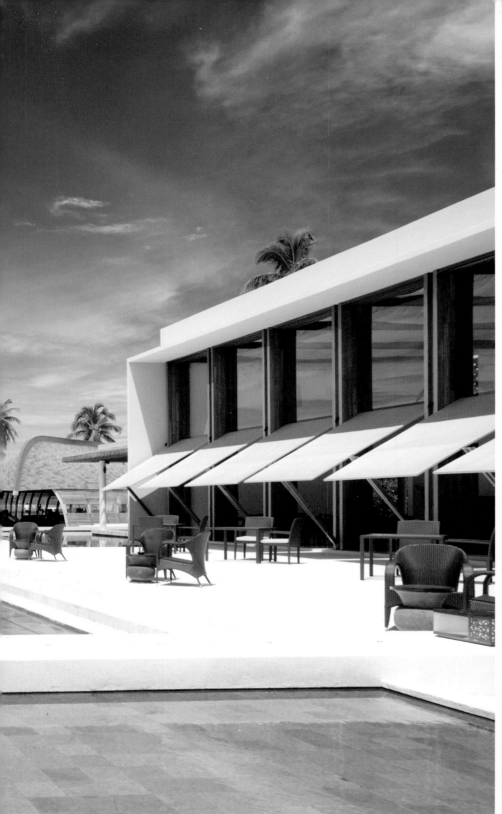

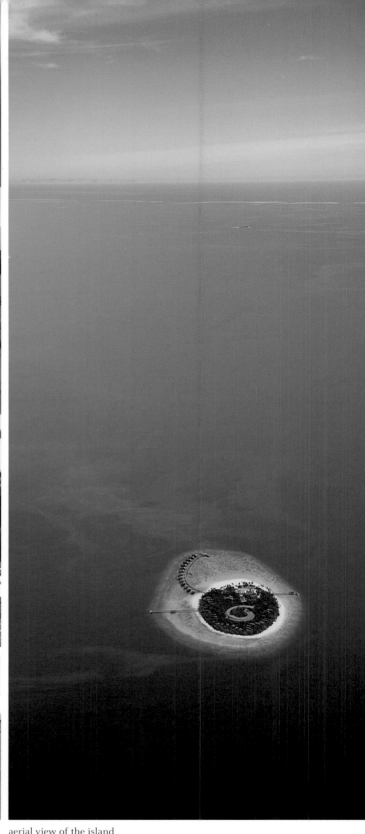

aerial view of the island

Park Hyatt Maldives Hadahaa

Hadahaa, Maldives

Architect: Chan Soo Khian, SCDA Architects
Location: North Huvadhoo, Gaafu Alifu Atoll, Republic of Maldives
Year of completion: 2009
Type of retreat: island retreat

Contemporary design with unique architecture, accommodating comfort and environmental sensitivity. The resort offers a great destination with an expanse of personal space. It was designed to minimize its impact on the environment and is the first project in the Maldives to be environmentally certified by Green Globe (now – Earth-Check) for planning, design and construction.

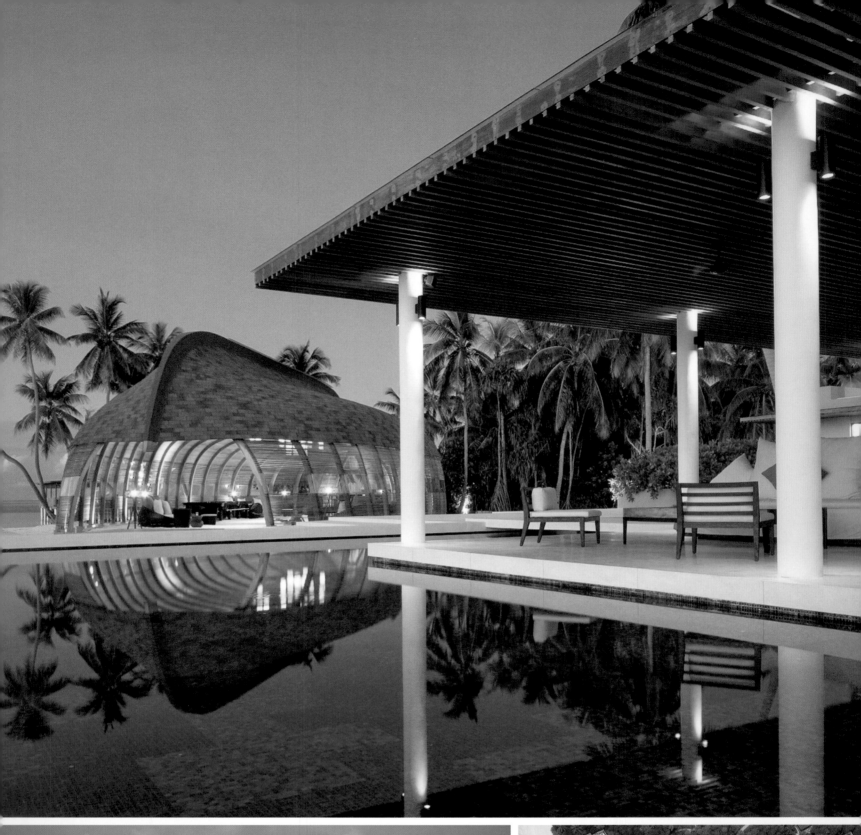

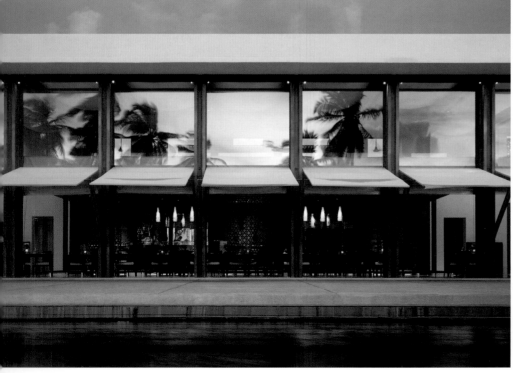

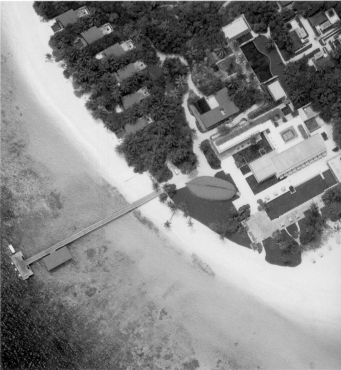

from above to below, from left to right: panorama view, dining room, aerial view

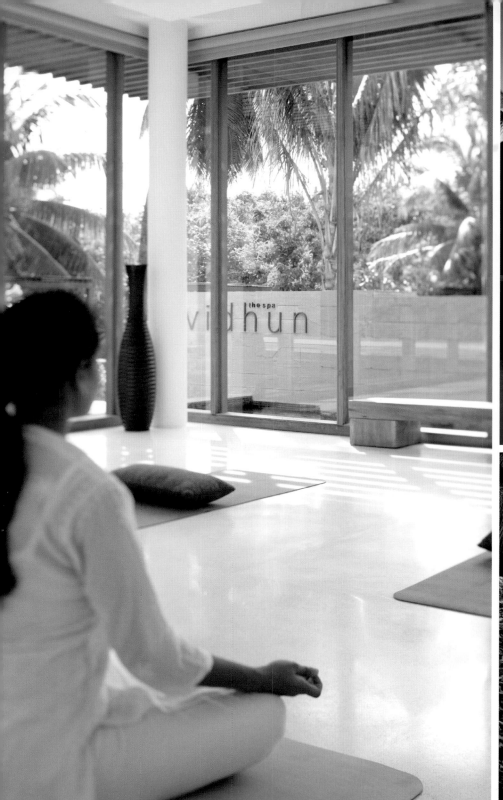

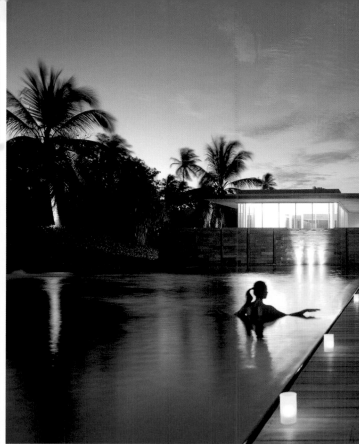

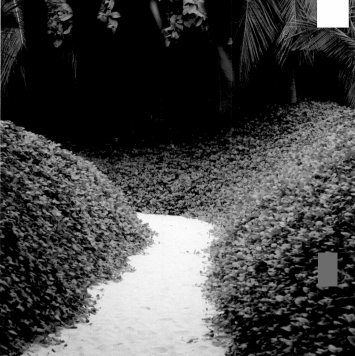

from left to right, from above to below: yoga studio, spa, path to the spa, floor plan

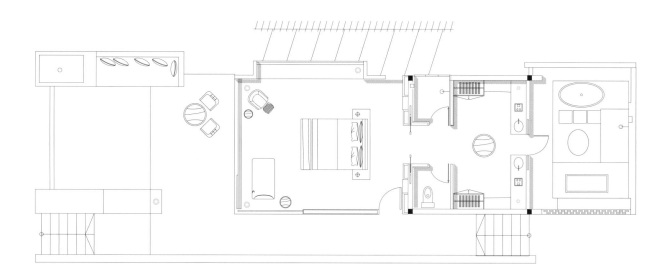

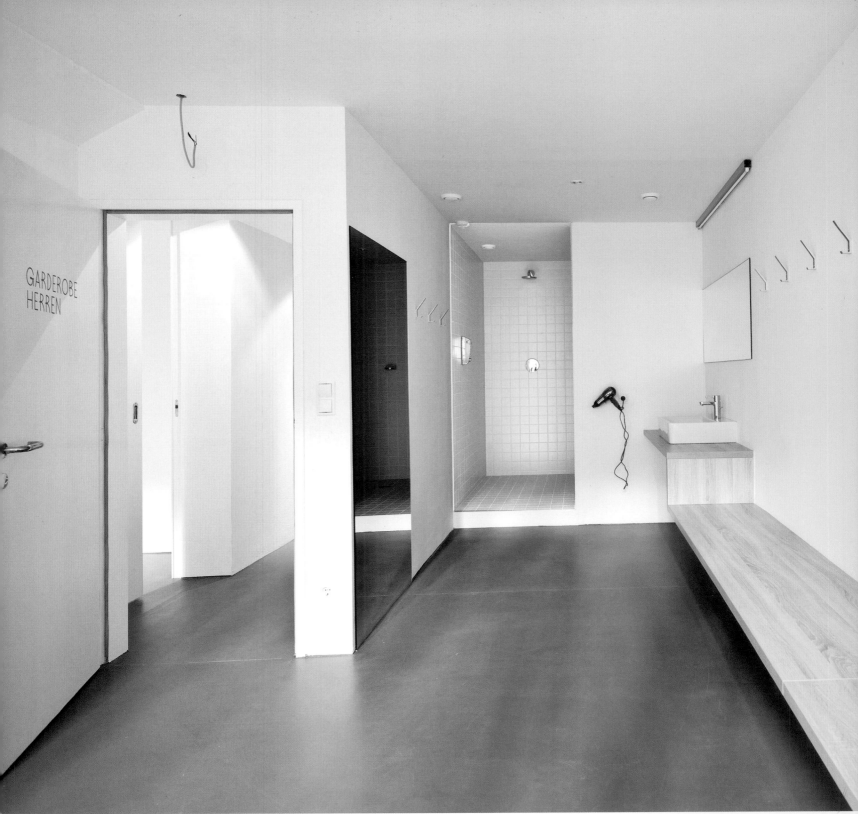

GARDEROBE
HERREN

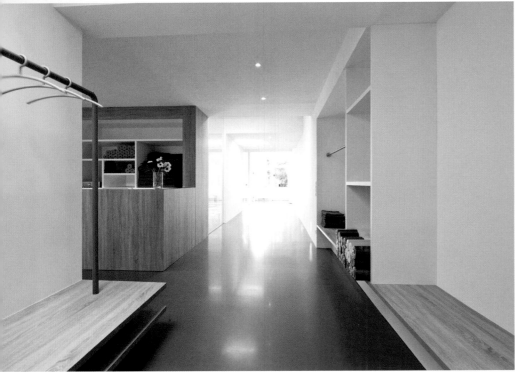

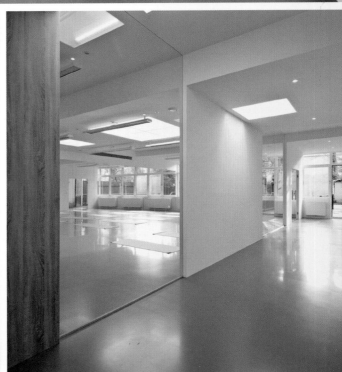

from above to below, from left to right: changing room, reception,
yoga room

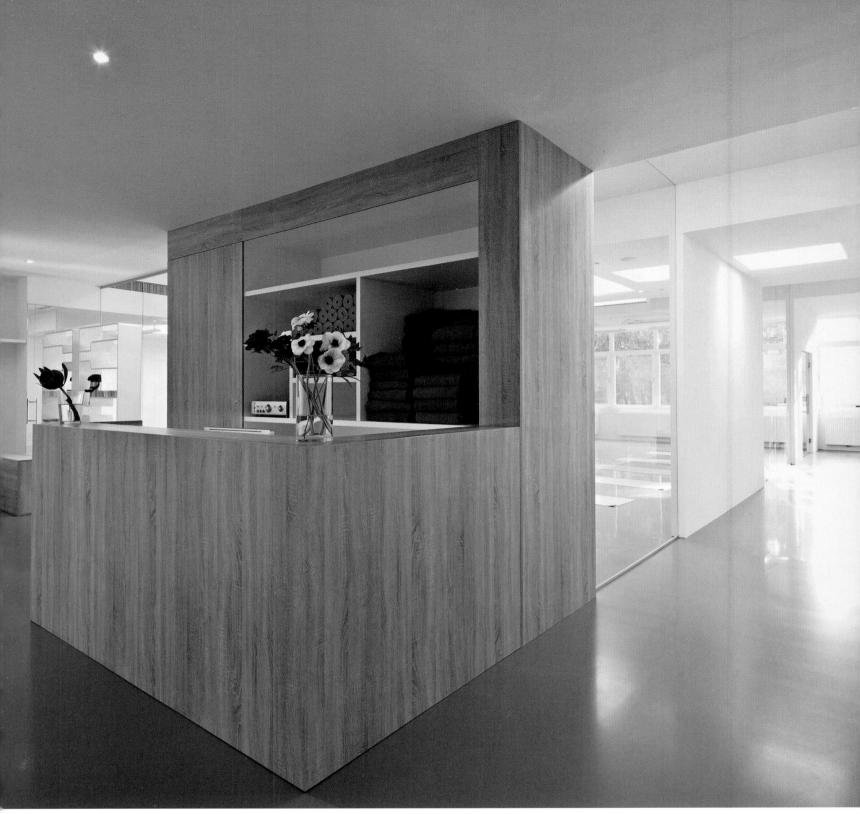

reception

Bikram Yoga Studio

Vienna, Austria

Architect:
PLOV Architekten
Location: Hietzinger
Hauptstrasse 9,
1130 Vienna, Austria
Year of completion: 2012
Area: 370 sqm
Type of retreat: yoga studio

The quartz grey floor running from the entry area to the basement provides continuity in the space, and highlights the customer areas. The material concept is augmented by a few pieces of wood furniture which tame the restless effect of the projections and recesses of the space while providing the needed warmth. Seating cubes and yoga mats contribute the color accents. The perspective from the entrance to the grass covered courtyard is preserved, while the wall constantly opening to the hotroom provides glimpses into the yoga events, allowing the room to appear expansive in spite of the separation. The basement is organized with just a few interventions. A rigorous color scheme highlights the restroom island which is surrounded by a circumferential path allowing the rooms to open up.

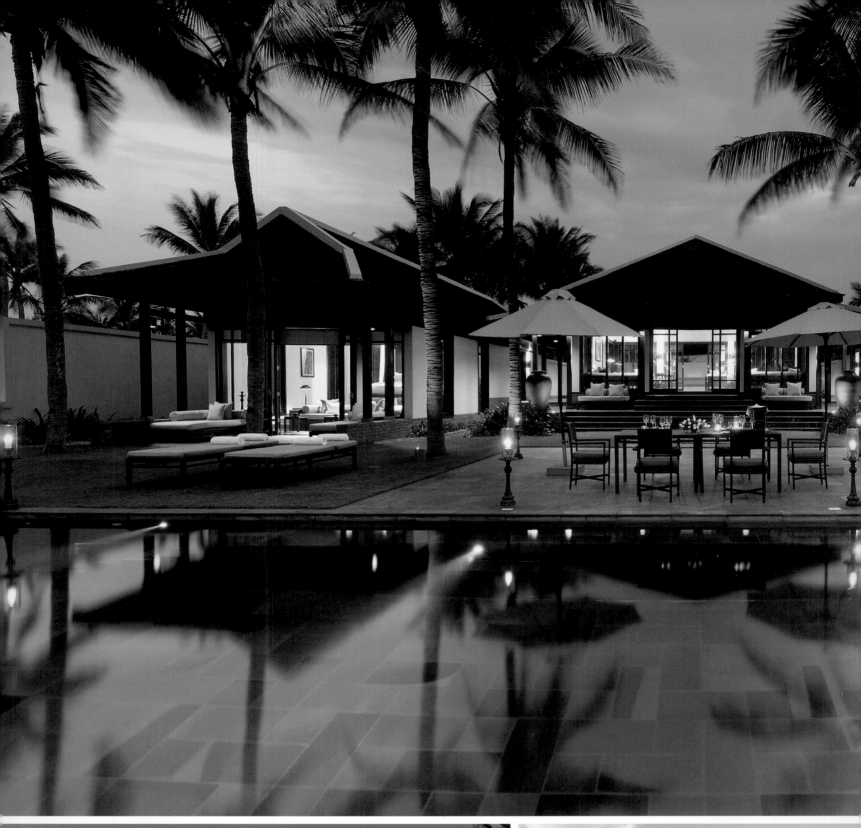

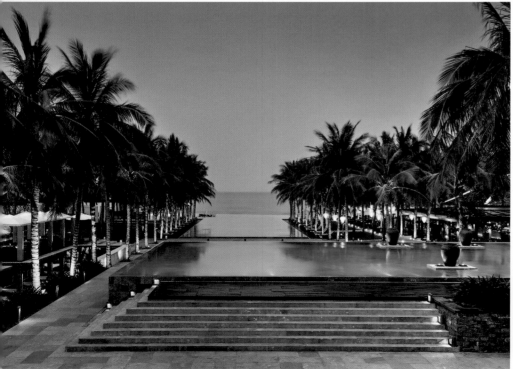

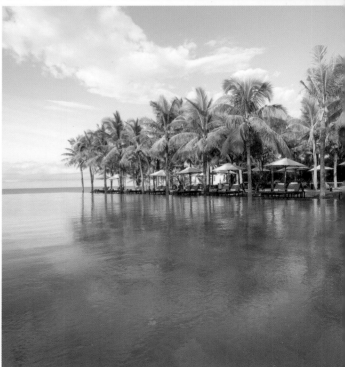

from above to below: bedrooms with pool, main pools with ocean view

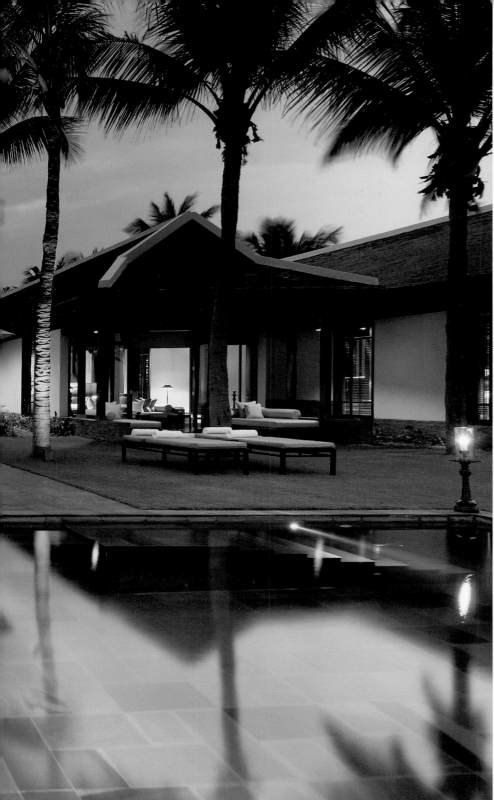

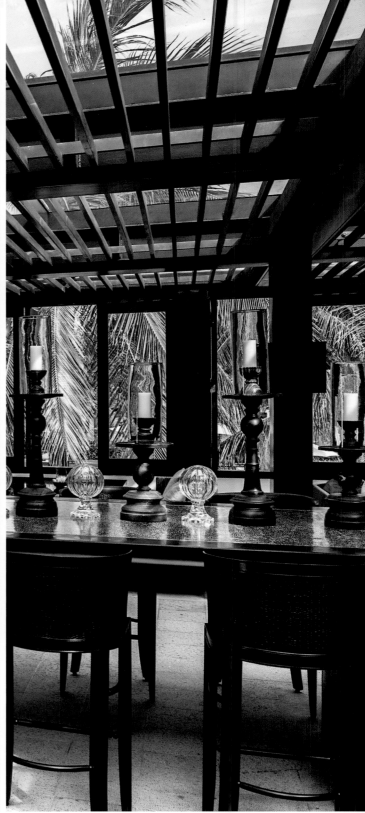

detail of the bar terrace

The Nam Hai

Dien Duong Village, Vietnam

Architect: AW2
Location: Hoi An, Hamlet 1,
Dien Duong Village Dien Ban
District, Quang Nam
Province, Vietnam
Year of completion: 2006
Area: 24,000 sqm
Type of retreat: 5 star hotel

In order to design the Nam Hai, the architects conducted research into Vietnamese vernacular architecture as well as into the more obvious Imperial architecture examples from the Hue and central regions. They decided in favor of a design based on the simple Vietnamese house, re-interpreted for a rich, modern Asian architecture. The core area is organized in a very controlled, geometric pattern of water and landscape, with the buildings carefully laid out in the overall landscape. They are presented as individual pavilions located at strategic points, with beautiful perspective views of the sea and the pools. The main pool is located directly on the main reception pavilion axis, with its length emphasized by the reflecting pond and the two other pools.

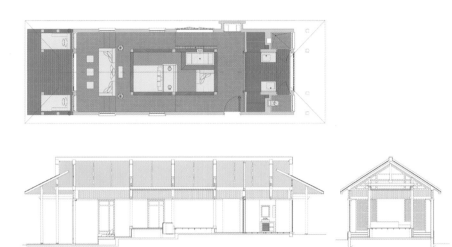

from above to below: floor plan and sections, main pool

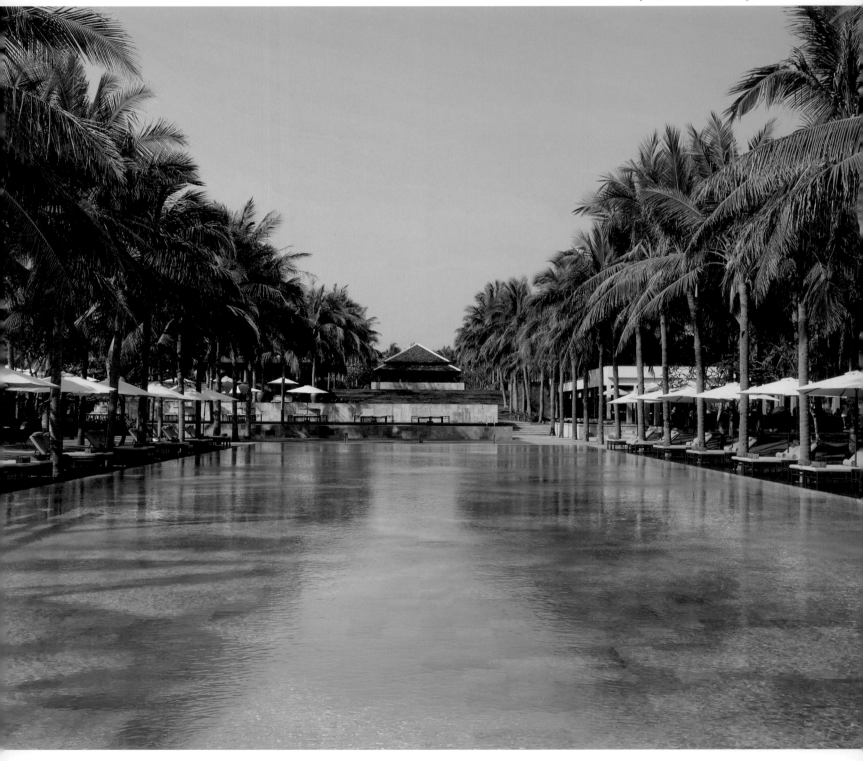

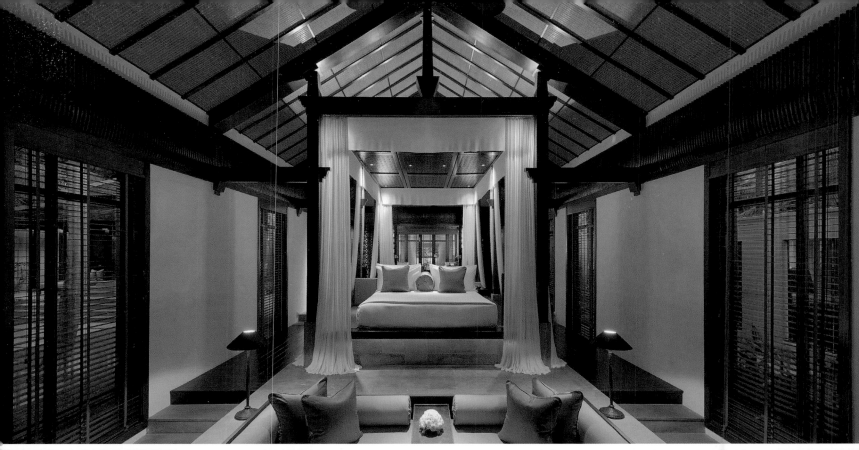

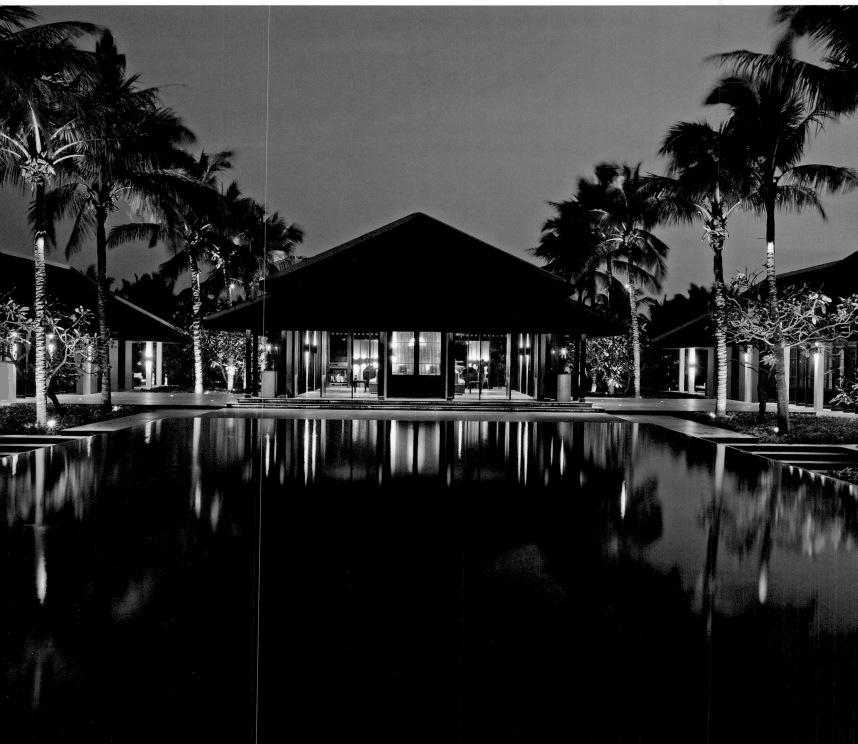

from above to below: bar entrance, lobby reception

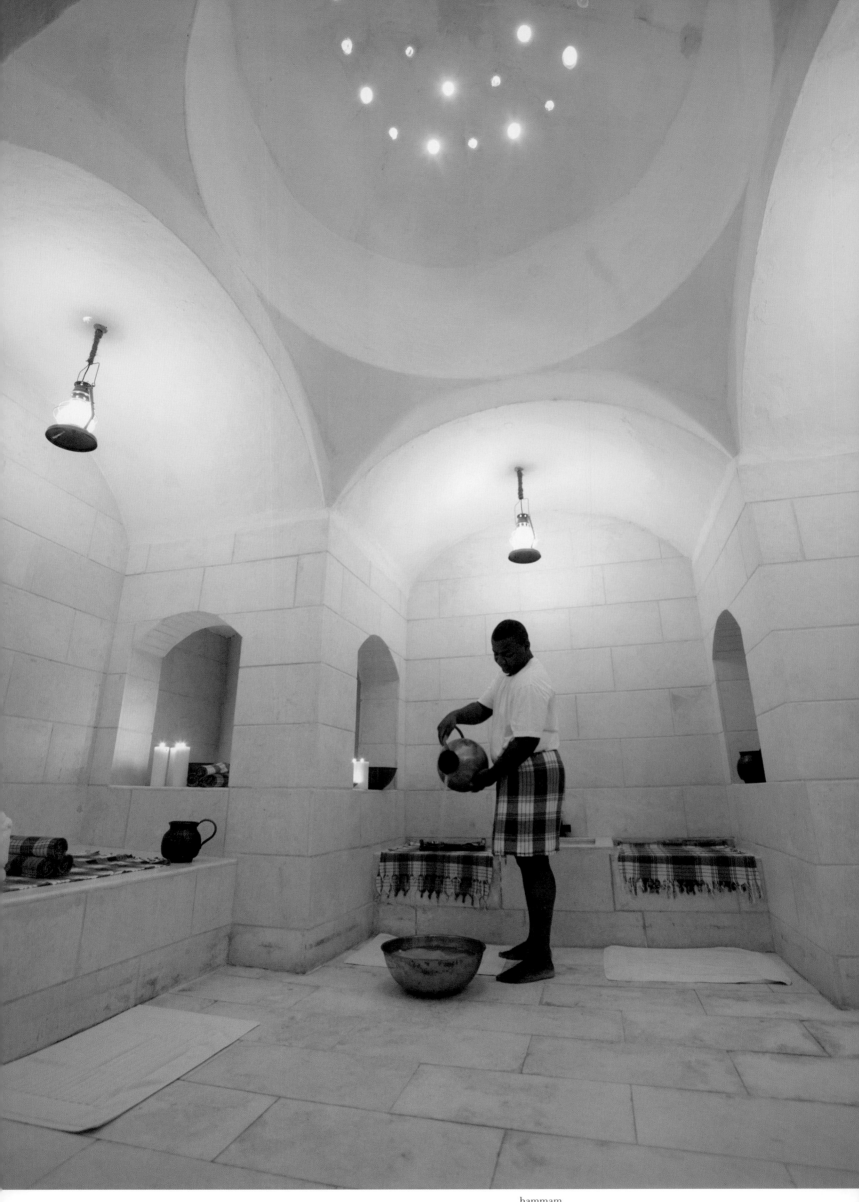

hammam

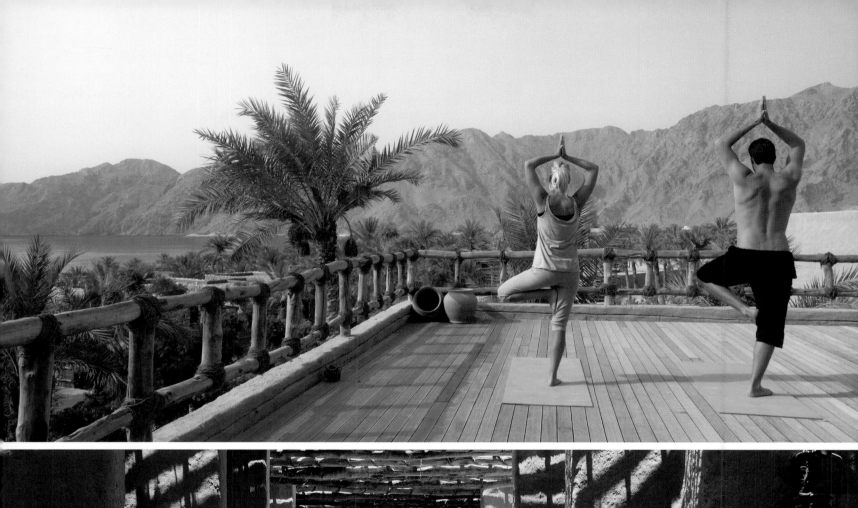

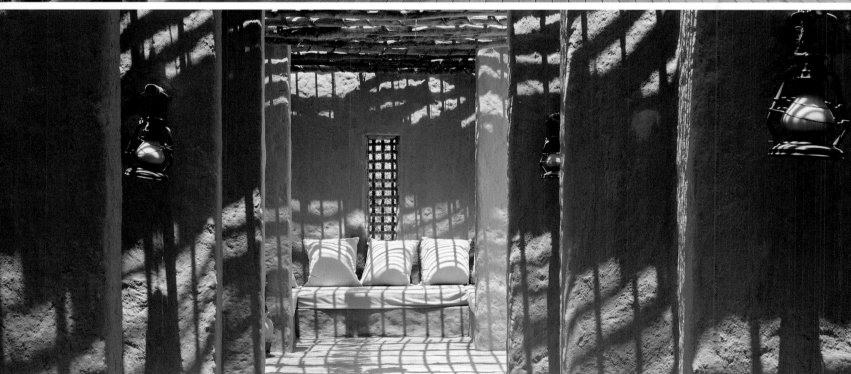

from above to below: people practicing yoga, entrance

Six Senses Zighy Bay

Dibba, Oman

Architect:
Al Araka Décor LLC
Year of completion: 2008
Type of retreat: hotel,
resort and spa

The eighteen acres self-contained Zighy Bay is set on 1.6 kilometers stretch of sandy beach ringed with rugged mountains and sea at the northern peninsula of Musandam. It features some of the most beautiful sandy beaches of Zighy Bay, with a temperate summer and winter climate. It includes the award-winning Six Senses Spa and Wellness Centre spanning more than 1,900 square meters. As the first Six Senses resort in Middle East, Six Senses Zighy Bay blends exceptional guest experiences with a unique style – authentic, personal, and adapted seamlessly to Middle Eastern and especially Omani cultures, in sustainable and harmonious individual surroundings.

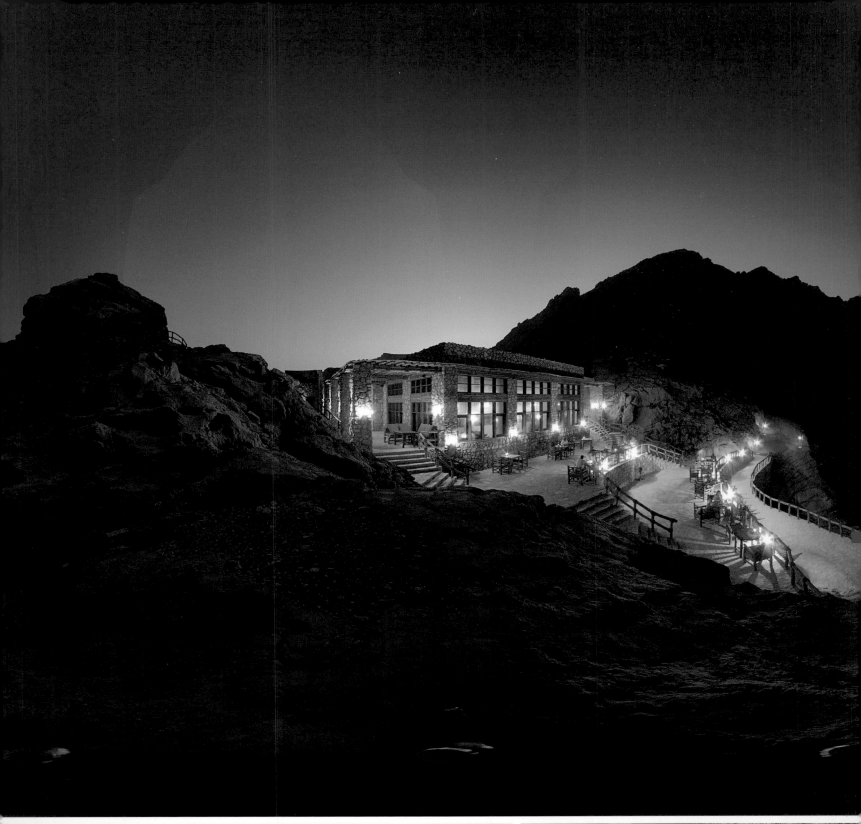

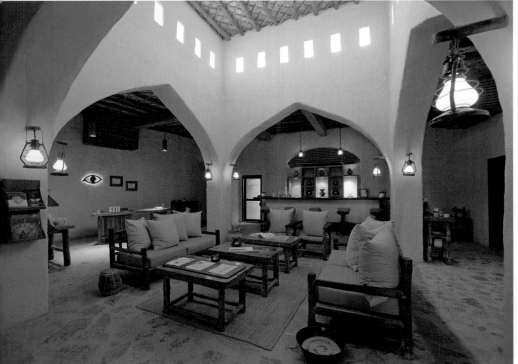

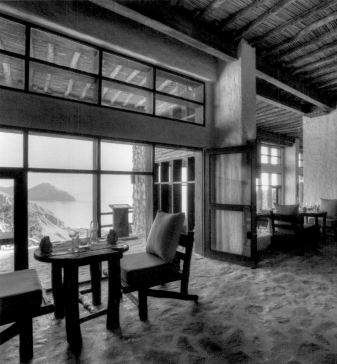

from above to below, from left to right: overview at night, spa reception, interior daylight

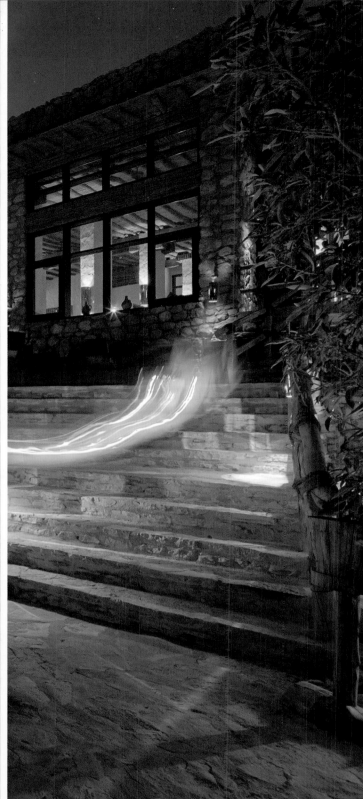

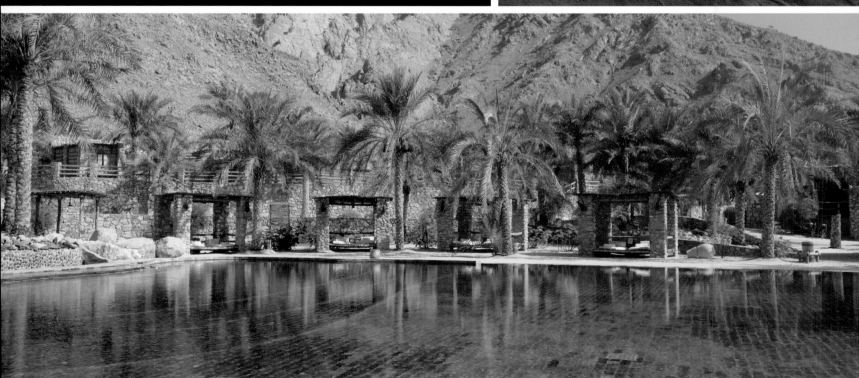

from above to below: terrace, main pool

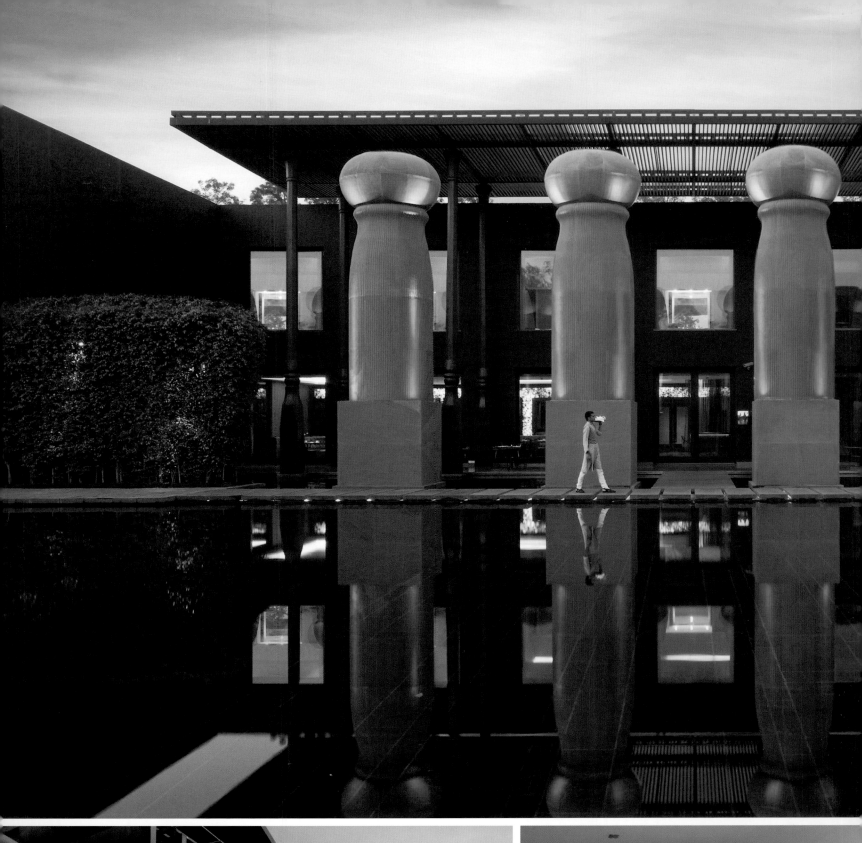

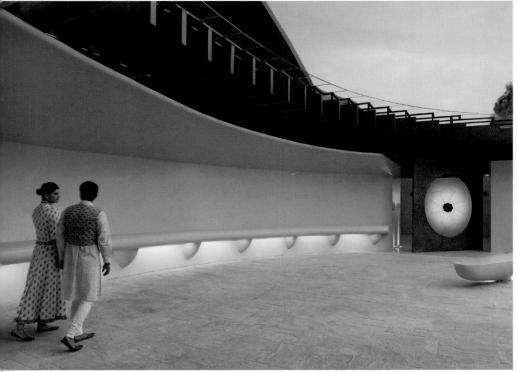

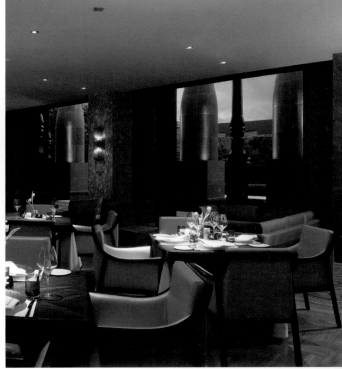

from above to below, from left to right: entrance area, arrival court, restaurant

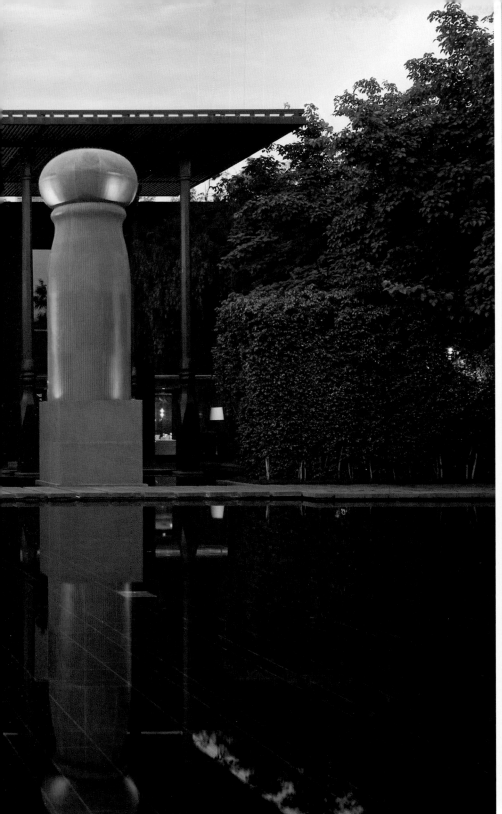

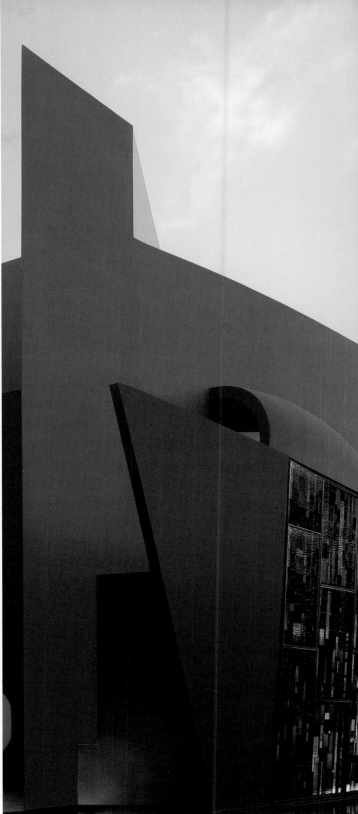

exterior view

Dusit Devarana

New Delhi, India

Architect: Bunnag Architects
Location: Village Samalkha, NH-8, New Delhi 110037, India
Year of completion: 2013
Area: 30,350 sqm
Type of retreat: hotel & spa

Designed by Khun Lek Bunnag, the Dusit Devarana is set amongst eight acres of luscious greens encompassing more than a thousand trees and water bodies, regally columned verandahs, and elegantly understated interiors. It hearkens back to the royal lineage associated with the greatness that is Delhi. The architect was inspired by the Hindu philosophy of "five elements", from the sun inspired dials, the flower motifs, the soothing toll of the temple bells to the extended bodies of water criss-crossing the length of the resort. His vision to integrate, art, architecture and nature into a single space, truly comes to life at Dusit Devarana.

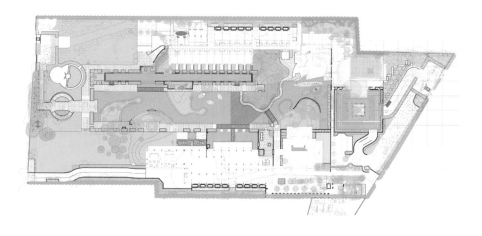

from above to below: site plan, bar, premier room

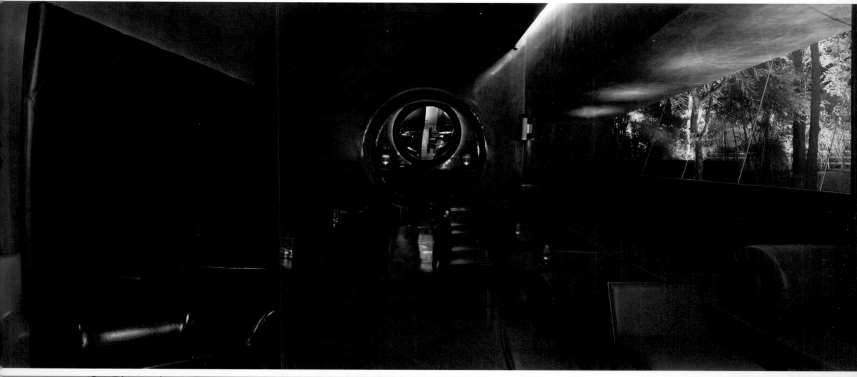

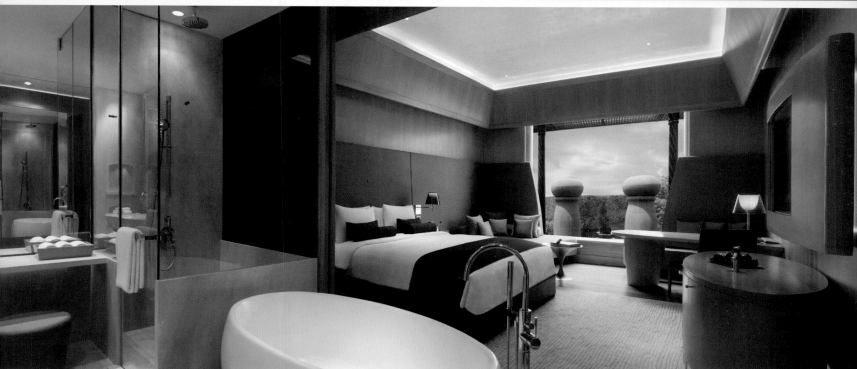

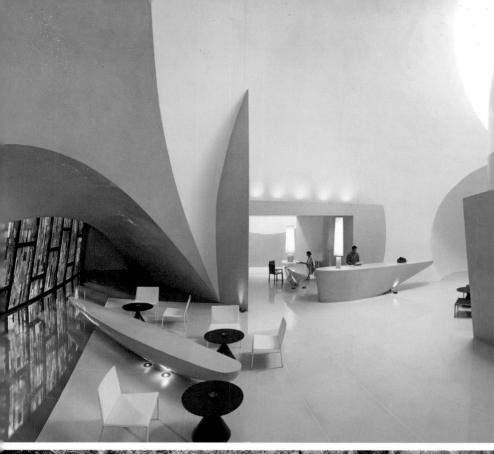
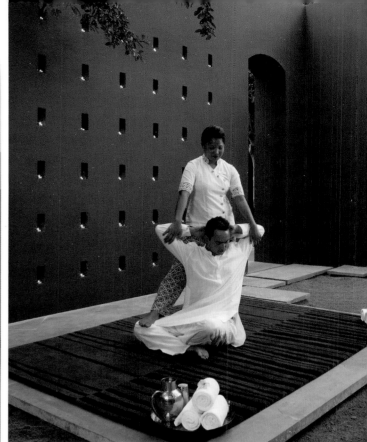
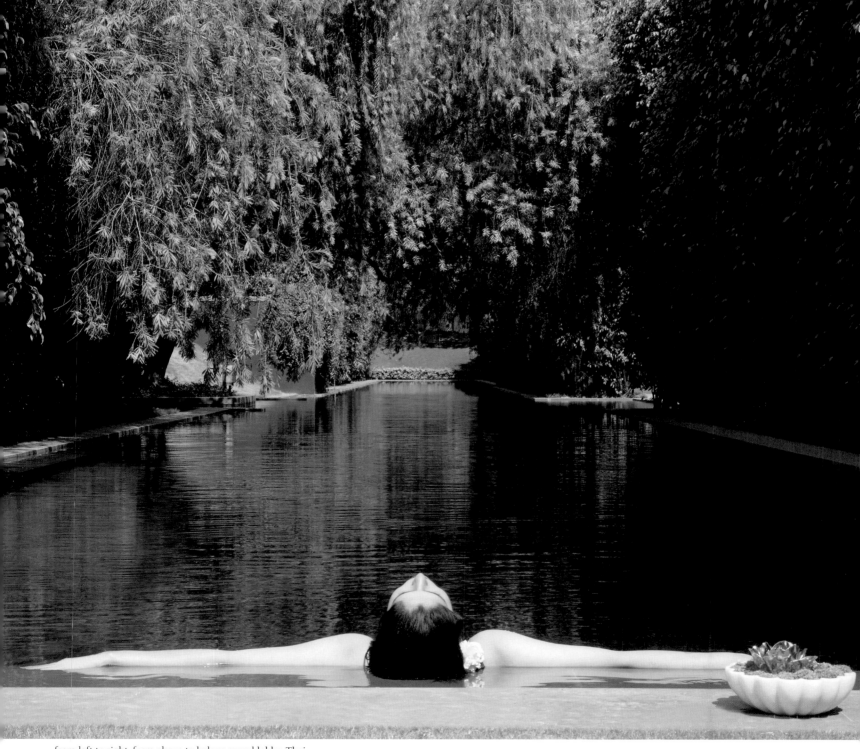

from left to right, from above to below: grand lobby, Thai
massage, pool

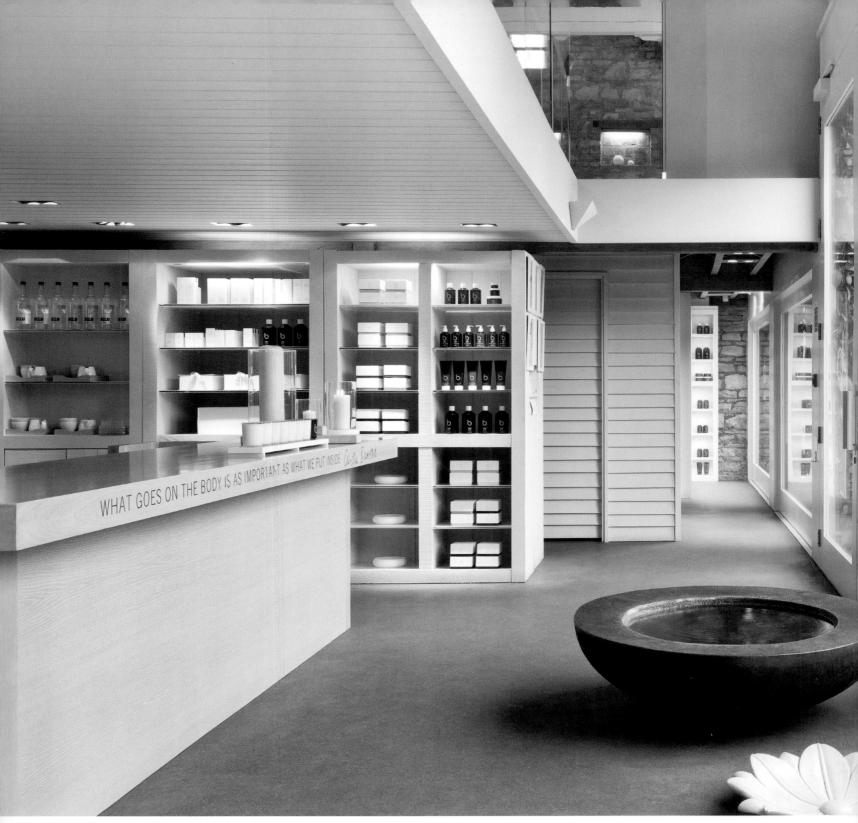

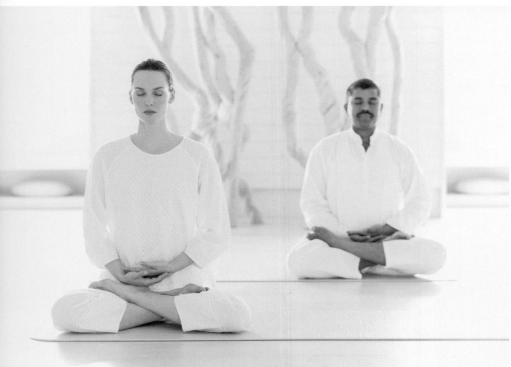

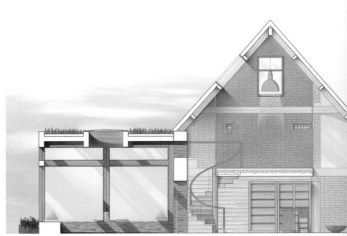

from above to below, from left to right: Haybarn entrance, people practicing yoga, section

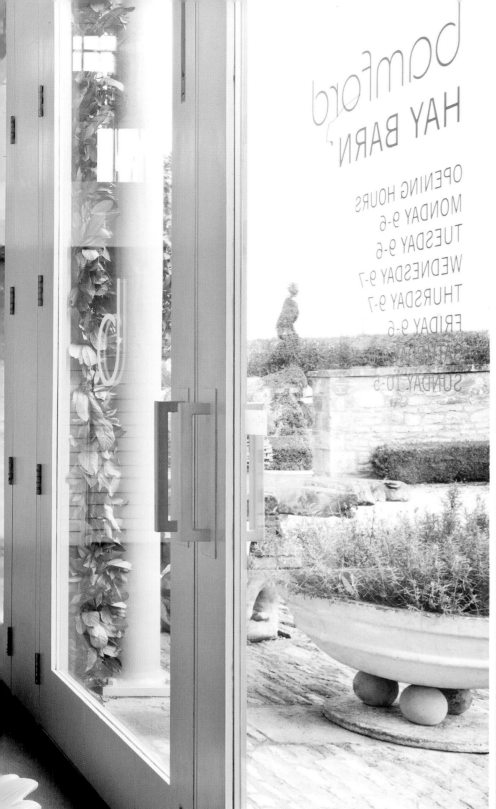

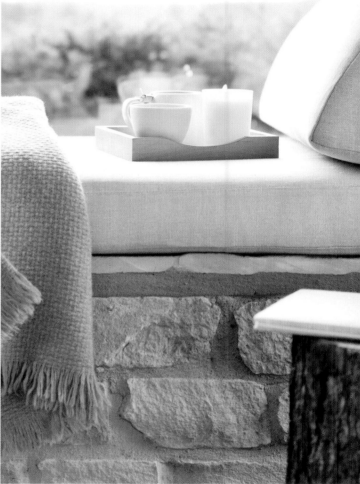

Haybarn lavender room

Bamford Haybarn
Day Spa

Daylesford, United Kingdom

Architect: Spencer Fung Architects
Location: Bamford Haybarn, Daylesford, near Kingham, Gloucestershire GL56 OYG, United Kingdom
Year of completion: 2006
Type of retreat: spa

Bamford is a way of life. The apparel company is inspired by nature to create collections for women that are timeless and nurturing. Bamford Haybarn in the cotswolds is a day spa that appeals to the mind, body and spirit. The holistic approach is based on the company's heartfelt connection with nature. A nourishing space for self-reflection and rejuvenation. The Haybarn offers yoga, Pilates, meditation, facial and massage treatments. The Haybarn is home to facilities that provide an environment of calm and tranquility. The individually crafted treatments use products specifically formulated for the Haybarn. The pure botanical products that cleanse, protect and invigorate are made from natural and organic ingredients certified by the highest standards of the Soil Association.

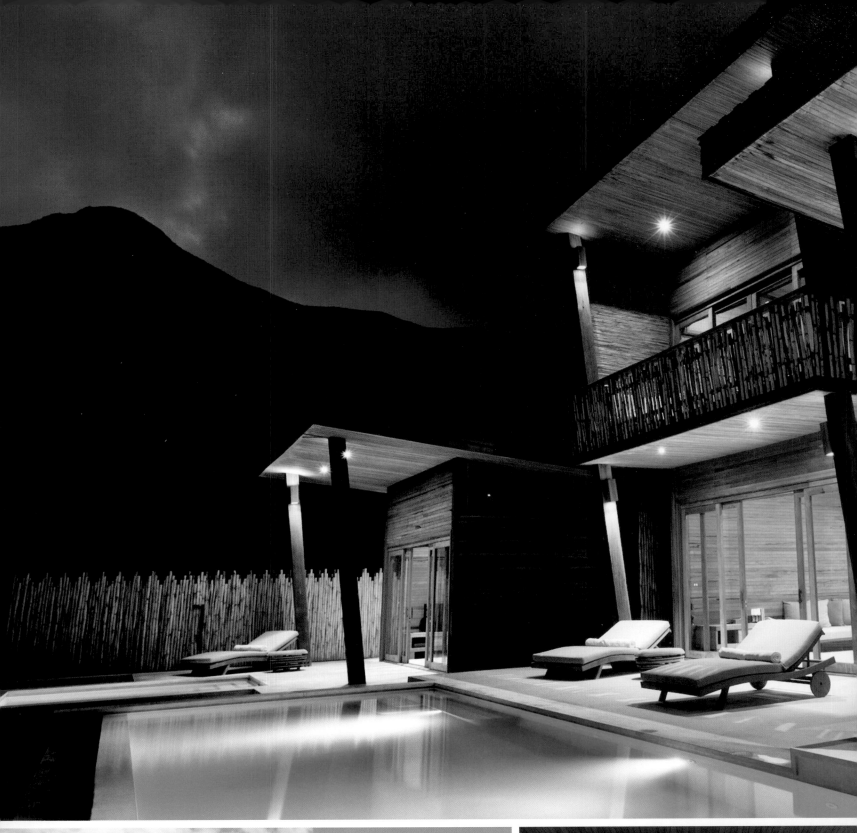

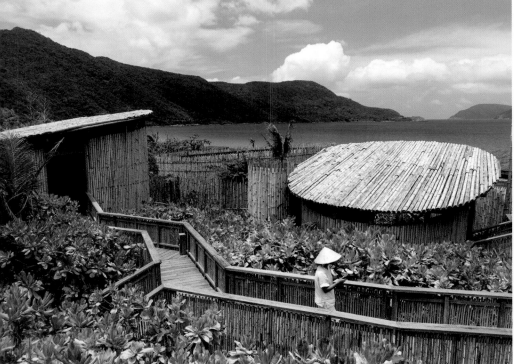

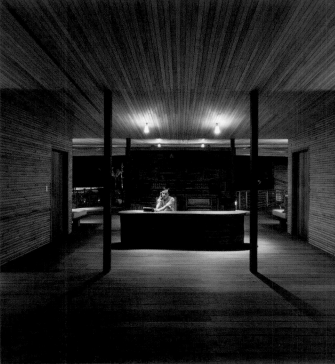

from above to below, from left to right: villa with pool, outdoor treatments rooms, lobby

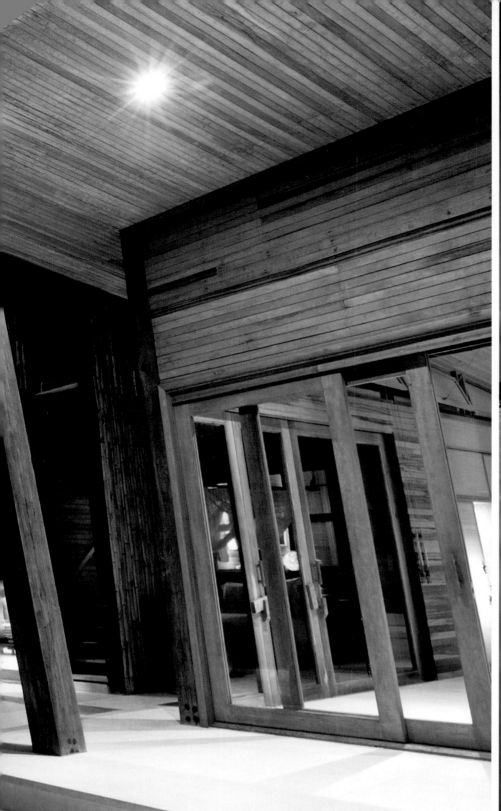
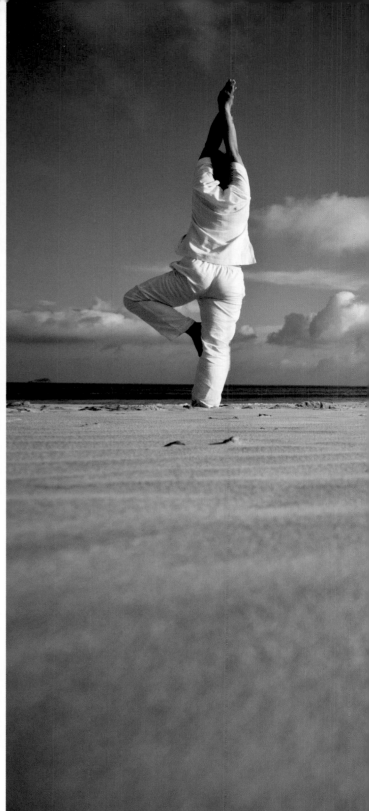

yoga on the beach

Six Senses Con Dao

Dat Doc Beach, Vietnam

Architect: AW2
Location: Dat Doc Beach, Con Dao District, Ba Ria Vung Tau Province, Vietnam
Year of completion: 2010
Type of retreat: hotel, resort and spa

Six Senses Con Dao is set in an area of outstanding natural beauty. The mansions sit along a mile of golden sand, looking out at the blue sea, the curve of the bay and the shelter of the darkly green forested Lò Vôi (elephant) mountain. The contemporary architecture of the resort has been designed to blend in with the natural surroundings and built according to Six Senses Hotels Resorts Spas' total commitment to the environment with natural, reclaimed, and sustainable materials. The heart of the resort has been designed to resemble a traditional Vietnamese fishing village and marketplace. Much reclaimed teak has been used, including more than a thousand antique wooden panels. A wooden bridge leads across a stream to the rolling sand dunes to the mansions and spa on the beach.

139

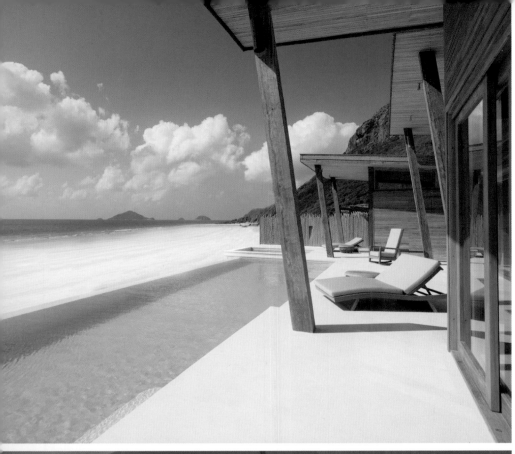

from above to below, from left to right: villa with pool, bedroom with ocean view, massage at Six Senses Spa

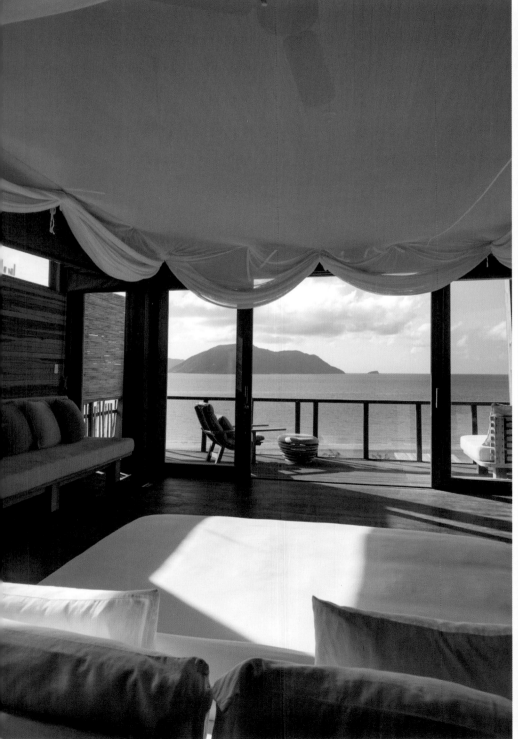

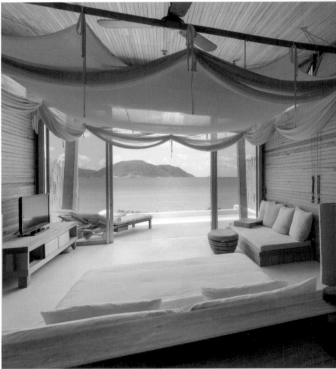

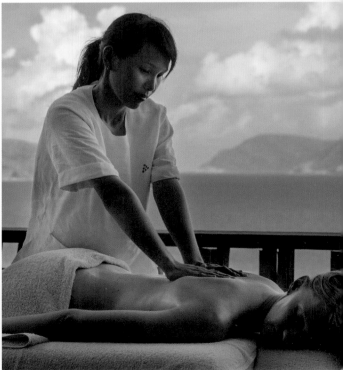

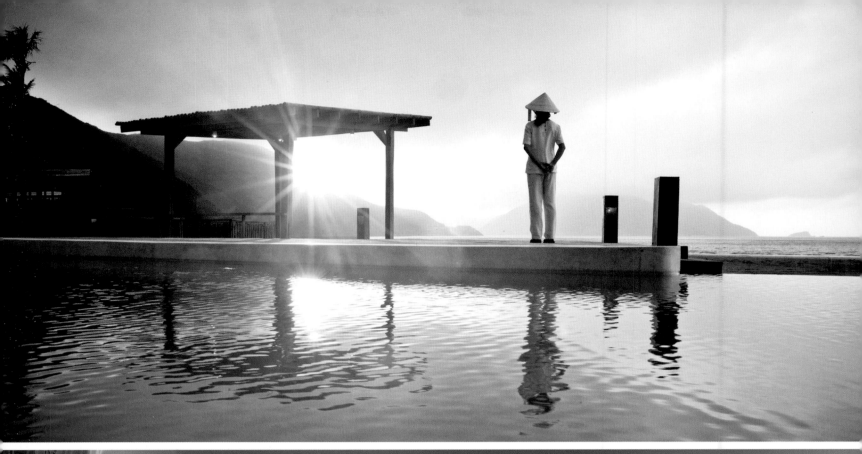

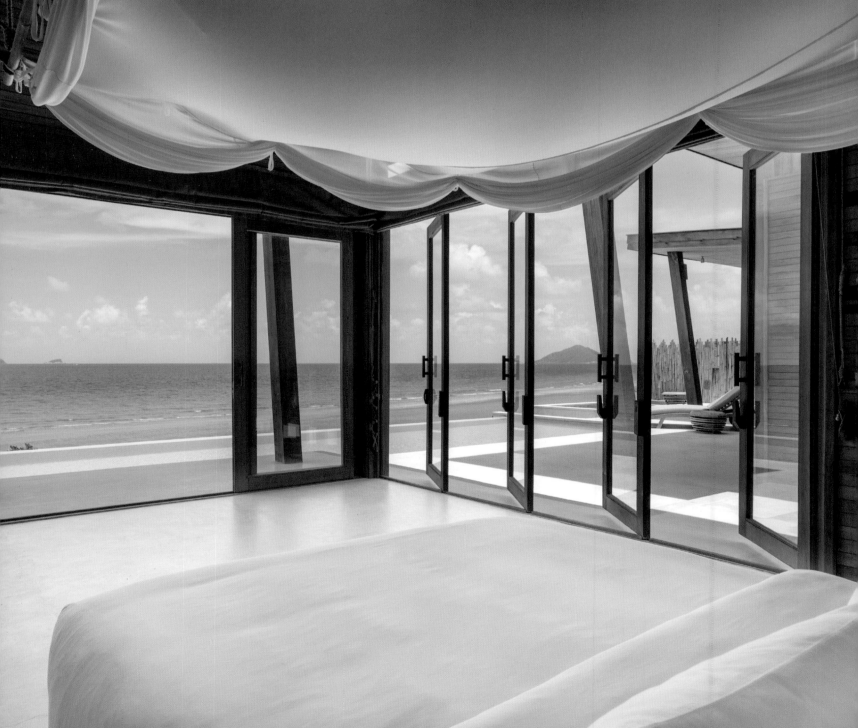

from above to below: main swimming pool, master bedroom

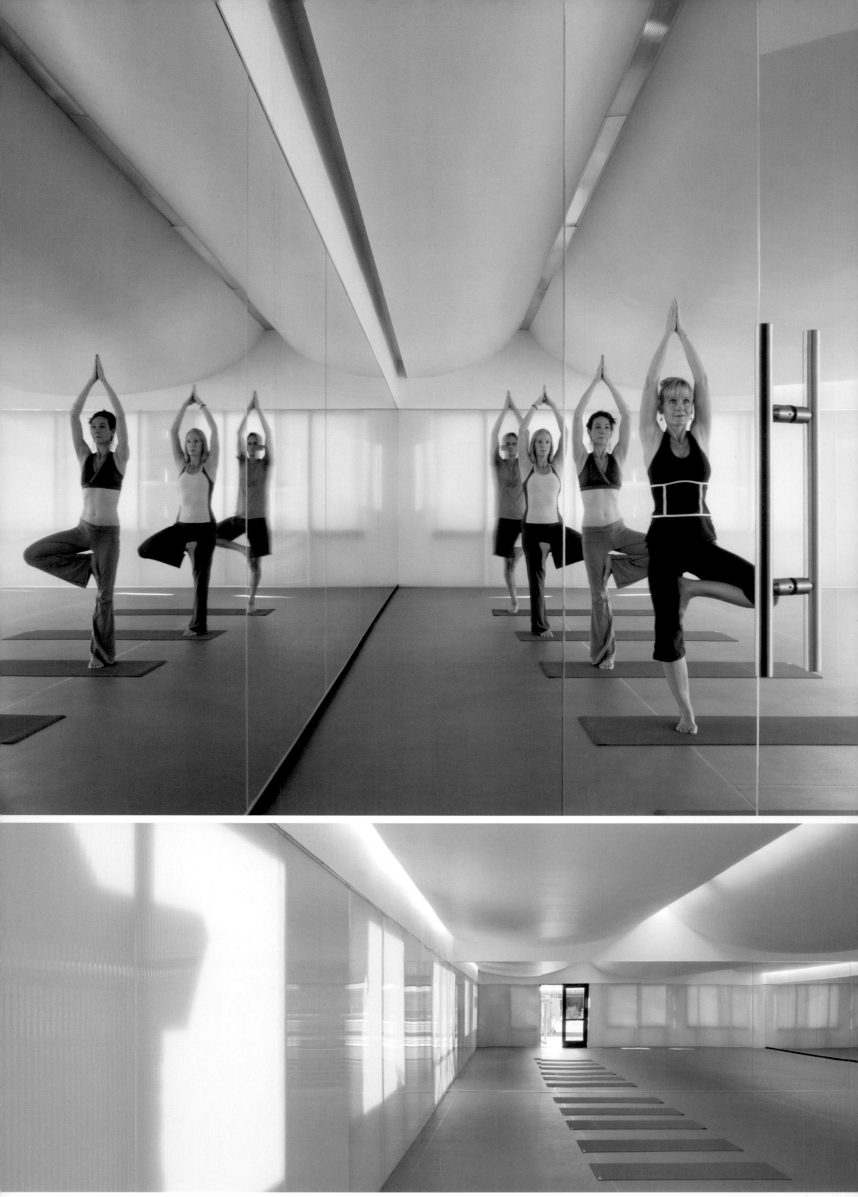

from above to below: people practicing yoga, yoga studio

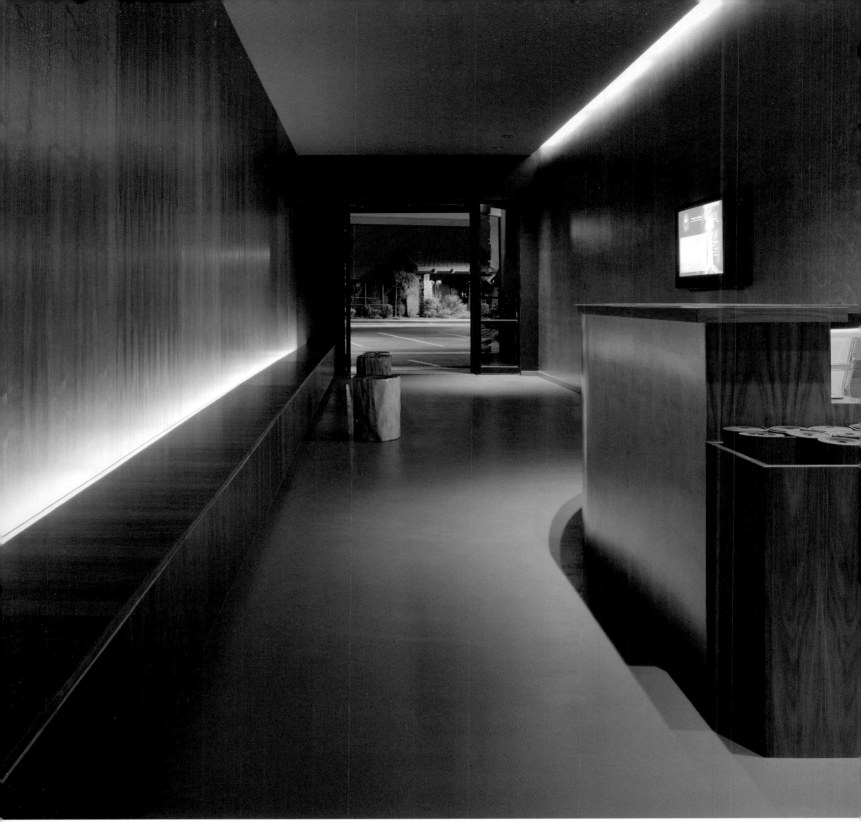

reception area

Yoga Deva
Gilbert, USA

Architect: blank studio architecture + design
Location: 2680 South Val Vista Drive, Building N.8 Suite 143, Gilbert, AZ 85295, USA
Year of completion: 2008
Area: 2,800 sqm
Type of retreat: yoga center

Yoga Deva creates an internal sequence of spaces whose primary impulse is to remove the visitor from the exterior visual environmental conditions in every way. Sited within a commercial condominium complex, the building is surrounded by asphalt parking, minimal planted islands of non-native decorative vegetation, and other buildings that are nearly indistinguishable from each other. This new internal environment offers an architectural and sequential chiaroscuro to the external strip-mall type reality and prepares the visitor for inward meditation and contemplation. Various styles of Classical Hatha Yoga are taught at this studio, including "hot yoga" which is performed in a space heated to 105 degrees Fahrenheit to improve flexibility and enhance detoxification.

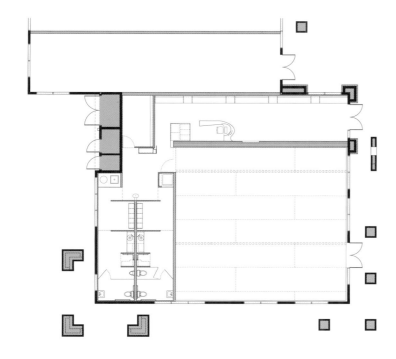

from above to below, from left to right: floor plan, reception, interior view

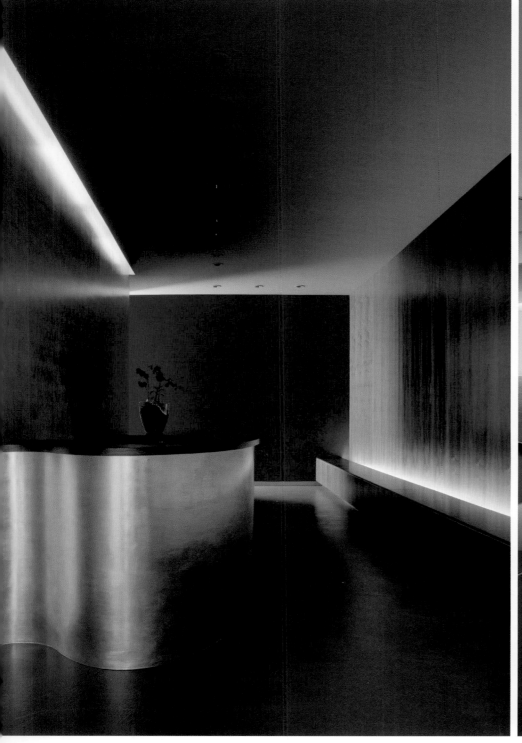

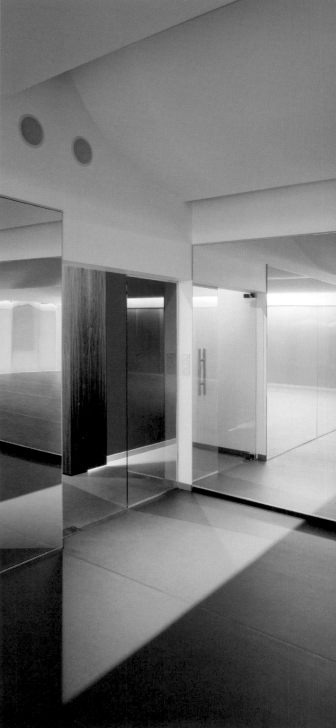

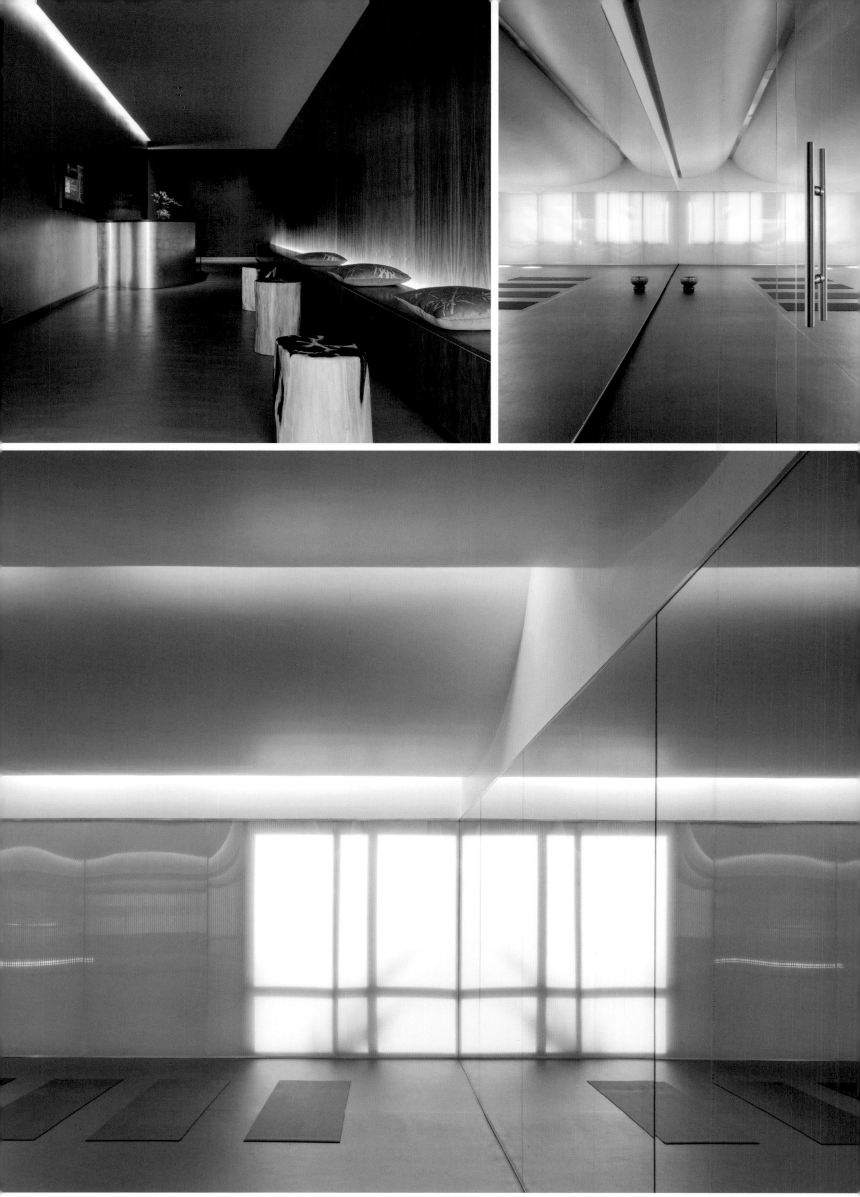

from left to right, from above to below: reception, entrance to
yoga studio from vestibule, yoga studio

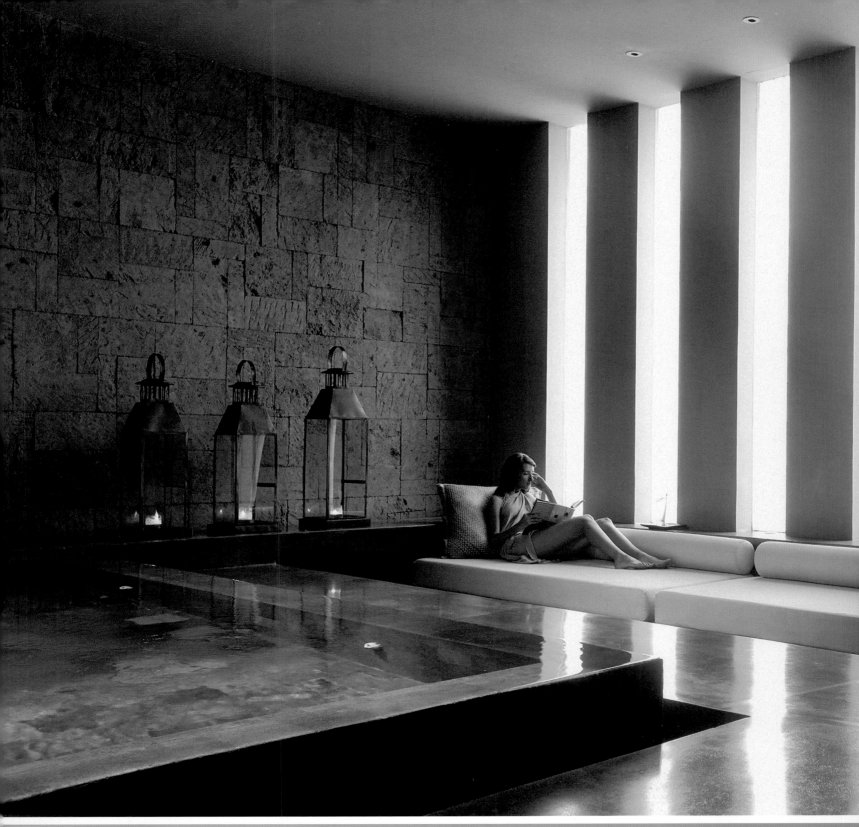

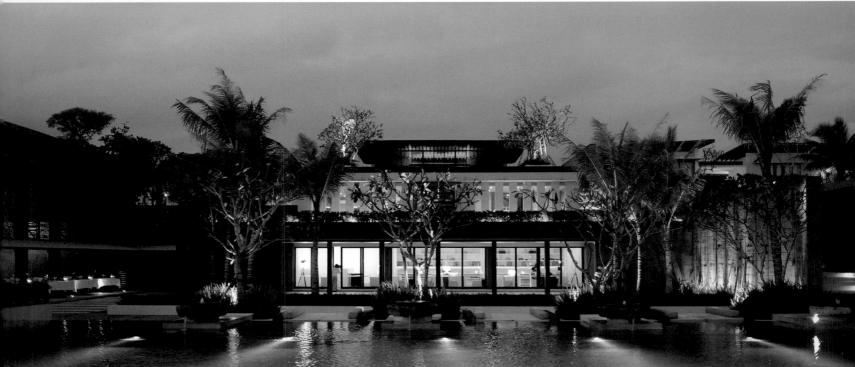

from above to below: reception area, main courtyard

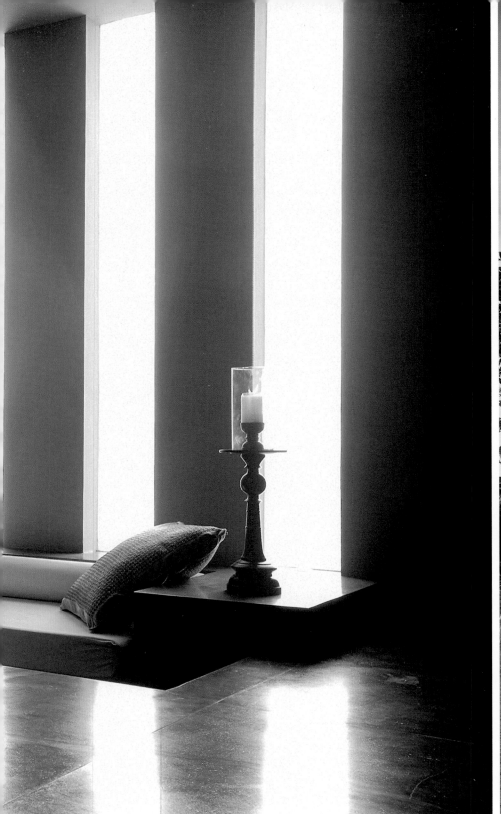

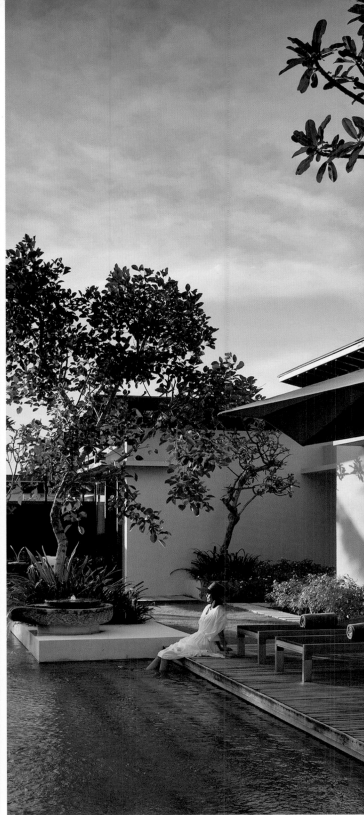

pool residence

Alila Villas Soori

Bali, Indonesia

Architect: Chan Soo Khian, SCDA Architects
Location: Banjar Dukuh Desa Kelating Kerambitan, Tabanan, Bali, Indonesia 82161
Year of completion: 2009
Area: 22,000 sqm
Type of retreat: resort

Alila Villas Soori is a design lover's paradise and a rejuvenating retreat. The resort comprises forty-eight mansions, all of which feature their own private pools and ocean views. Uniquely located in a small village in Tabanan Regency, Bali, Alila Villas Soori is the ideal destination for the traveler who wants a serene escape from a busy life. The unique location gives visitors access to three distinct geographical features — lush black sand beaches, mountains, and rice paddies. Tranquility and local elements guided the design of the architect, Soo Khian Chan. As guests navigate the resort, they'll notice indigenous stones and hear the calming sounds of water, an element which features prominently in the architecture.

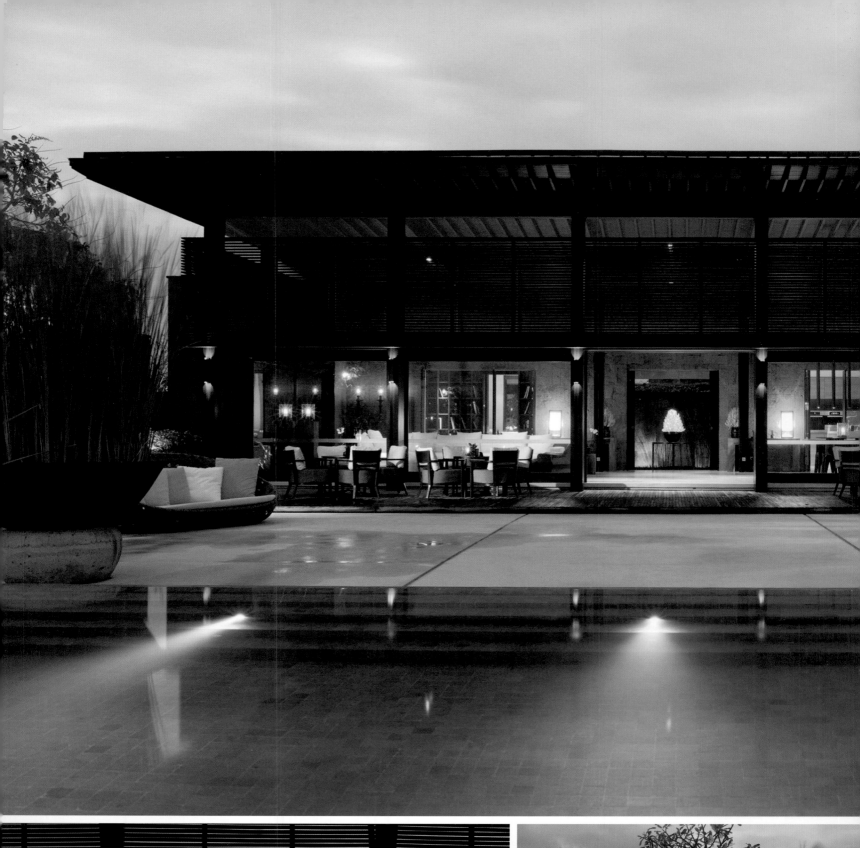

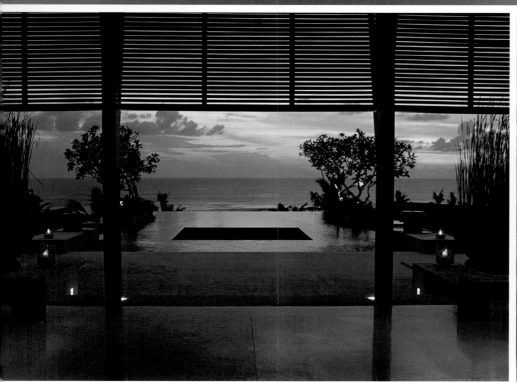

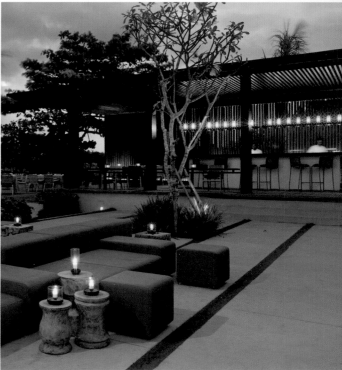

from above to below, from left to right: Soori estate, reception
pavilion, restaurant

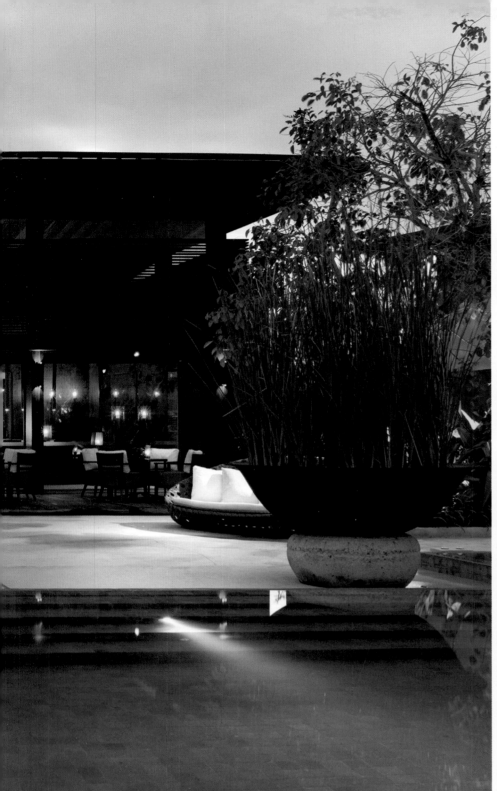

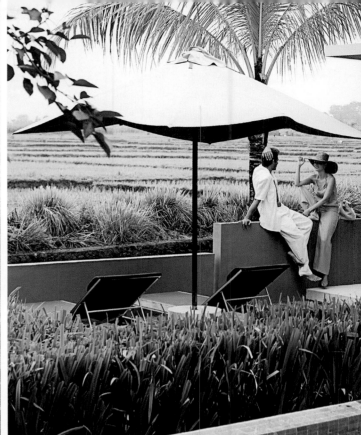

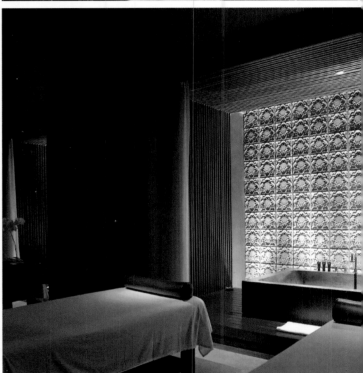

from above to below: mountain view, therapy room, floor plan
oceanfront villa

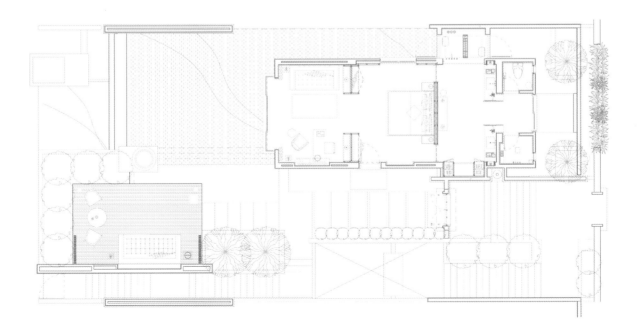

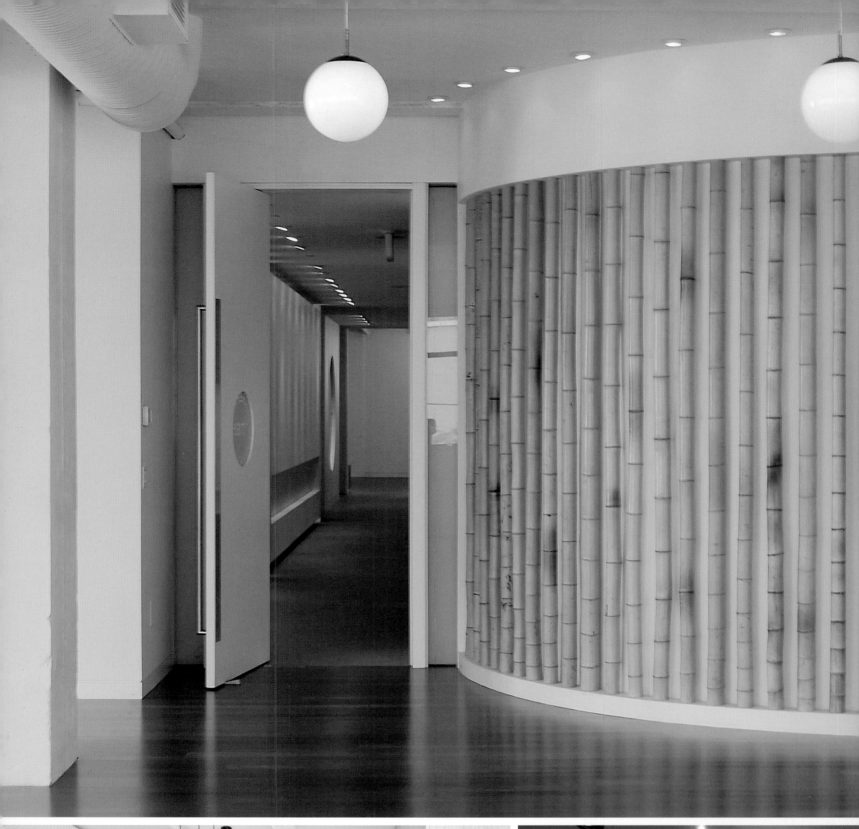

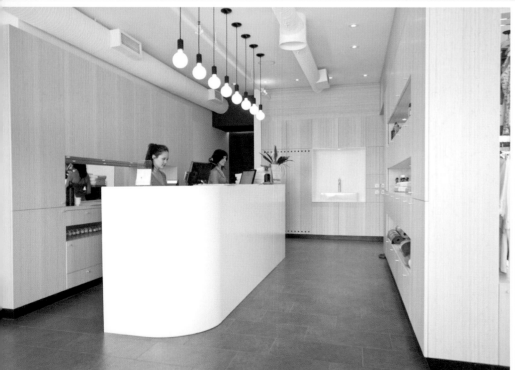

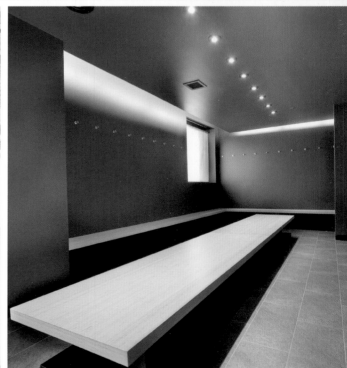

from above to below, from left to right: downtown flow – yoga room, reception area, women's changing room

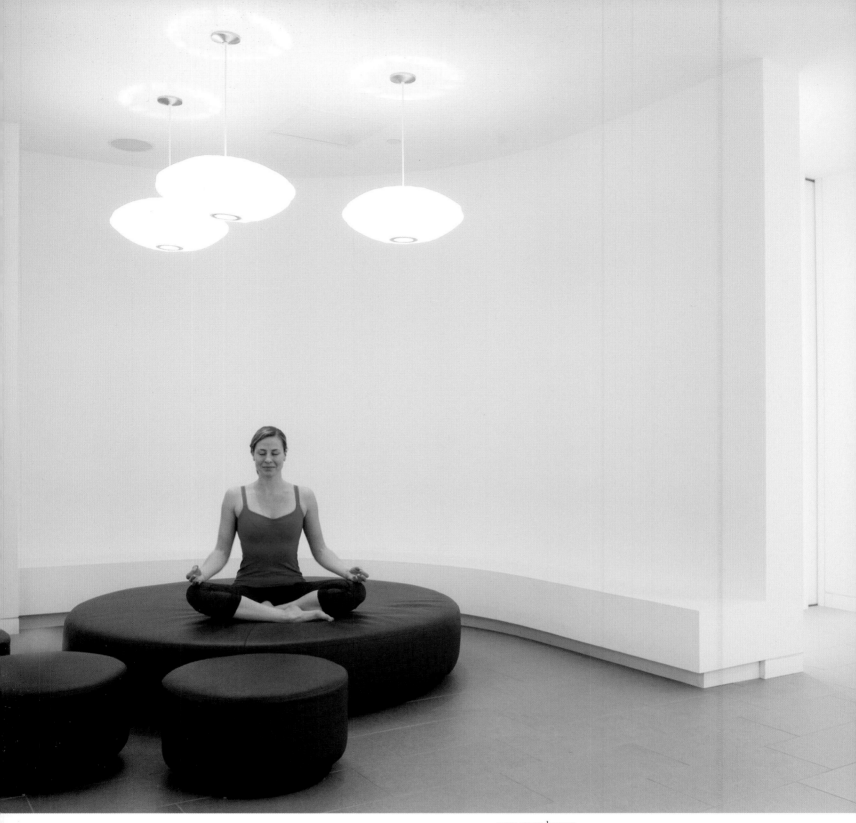

yoga room lounge

YYOGA – Studios

Vancouver, Canada

Architect:
Michel Laflamme Architect
Year of completion: 2008–2009
Area: 292–1,457 sqm
Type of retreat: yoga &
wellness center

The architect was asked to design multiple sustainable wellness centers focused on the practice of hot yoga. While using similar design elements like bamboo poles and bamboo built-in cabinets, each studio has a unique character that respects and reflects its environment. The main objective was to design spaces devoid of distractions, which would operate as some sort of "mental vacuum" for the users, in order to promote relaxation and focus. Three principles support that goal: the reduction of the color palette to white and grey, the use of materials that are haptically appealing and the elimination of distracting details, whereby the mind expands and the body reconnects with the regulating rhythm of breathing.

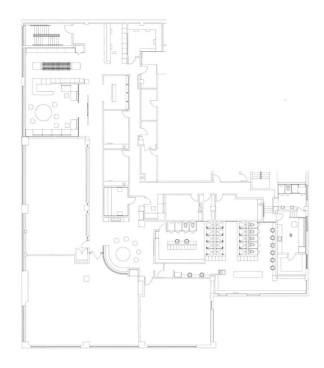

from above to below, from left to right: floor plan, detail of the wall, retail & water fountain, north shore elements – yoga room

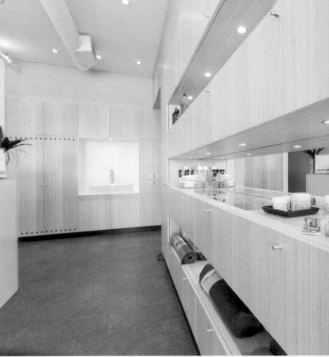

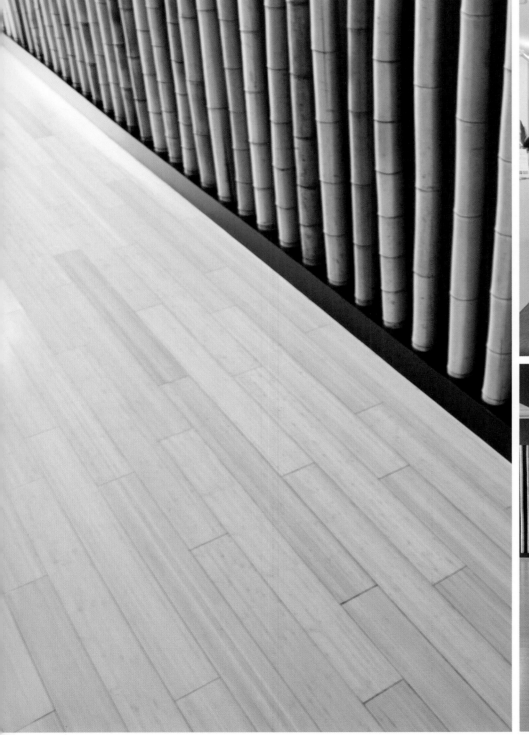

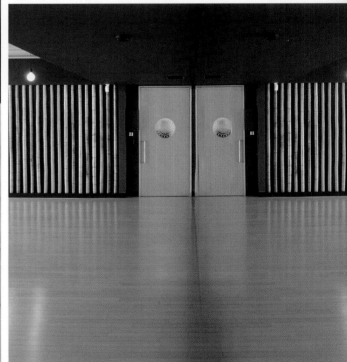

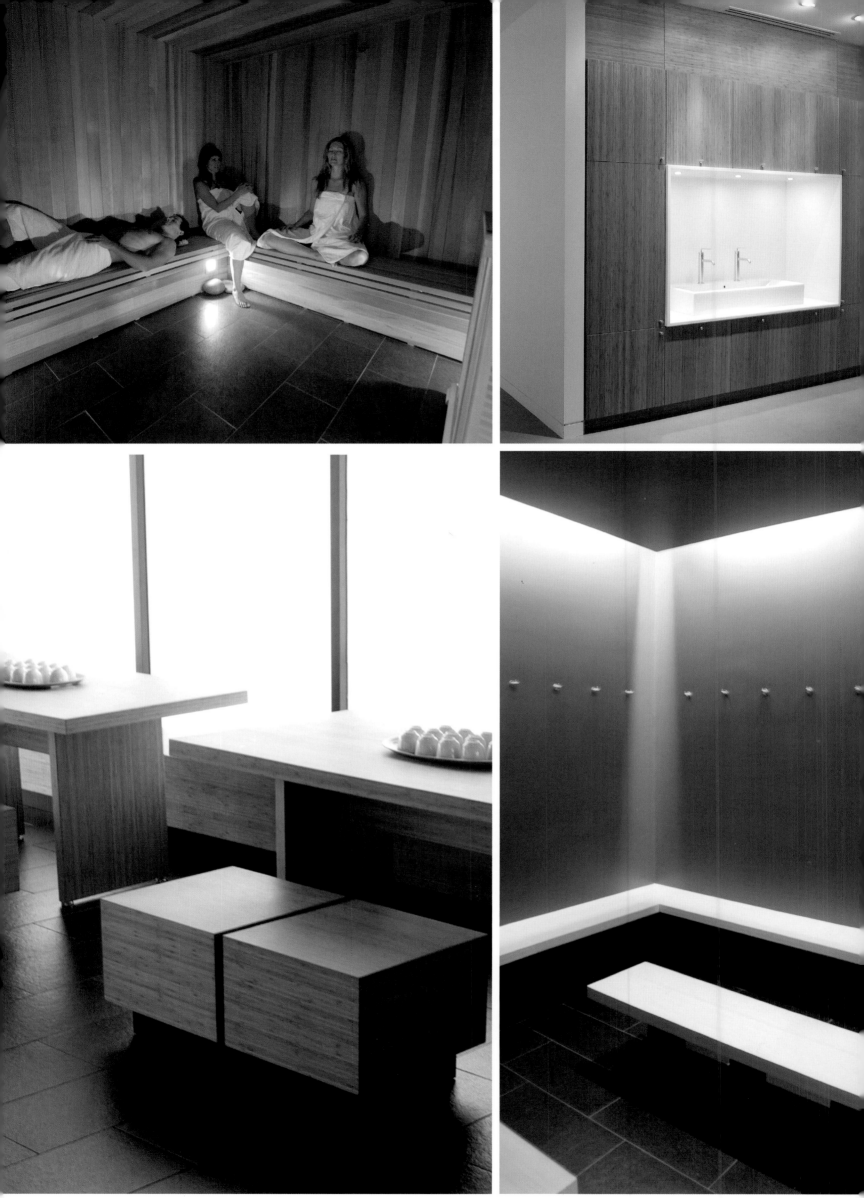

from left to right, from above to below: infrared sauna,
hallway, cool-down lounge, men's washroom

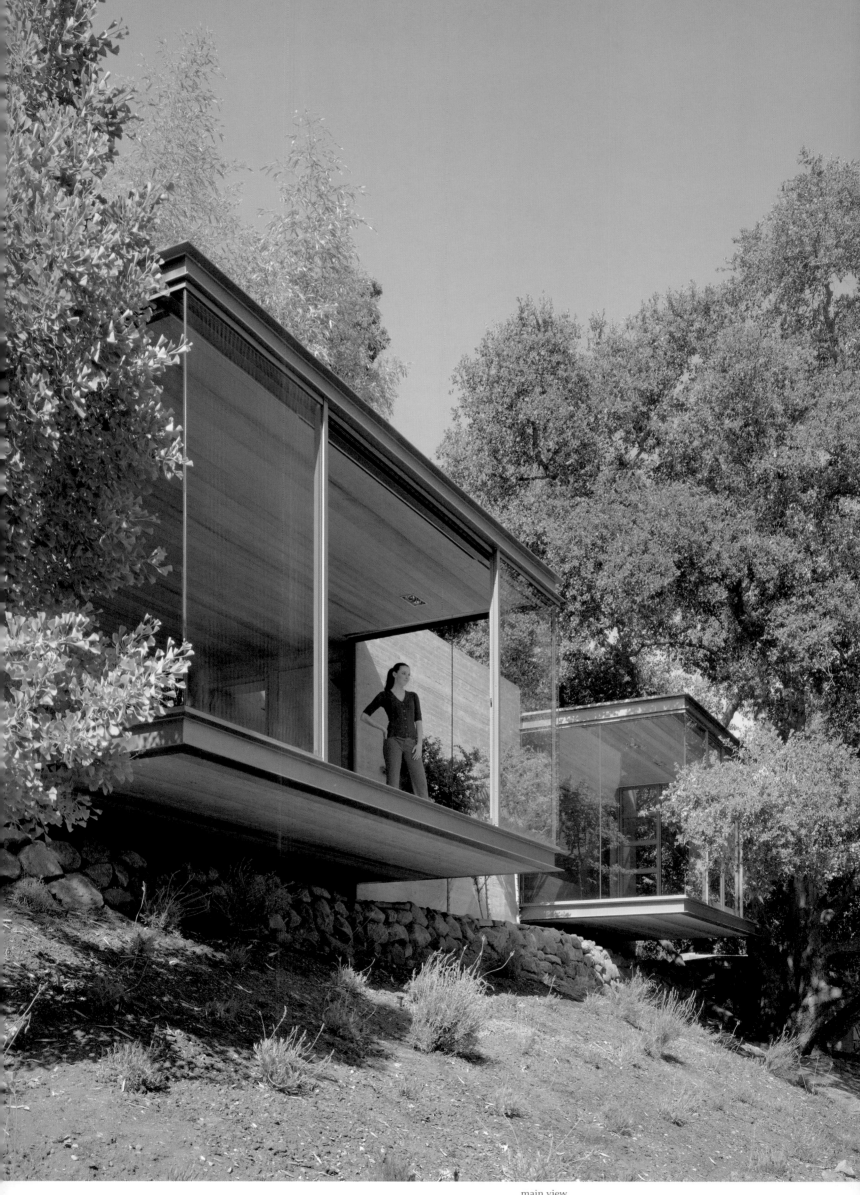

main view

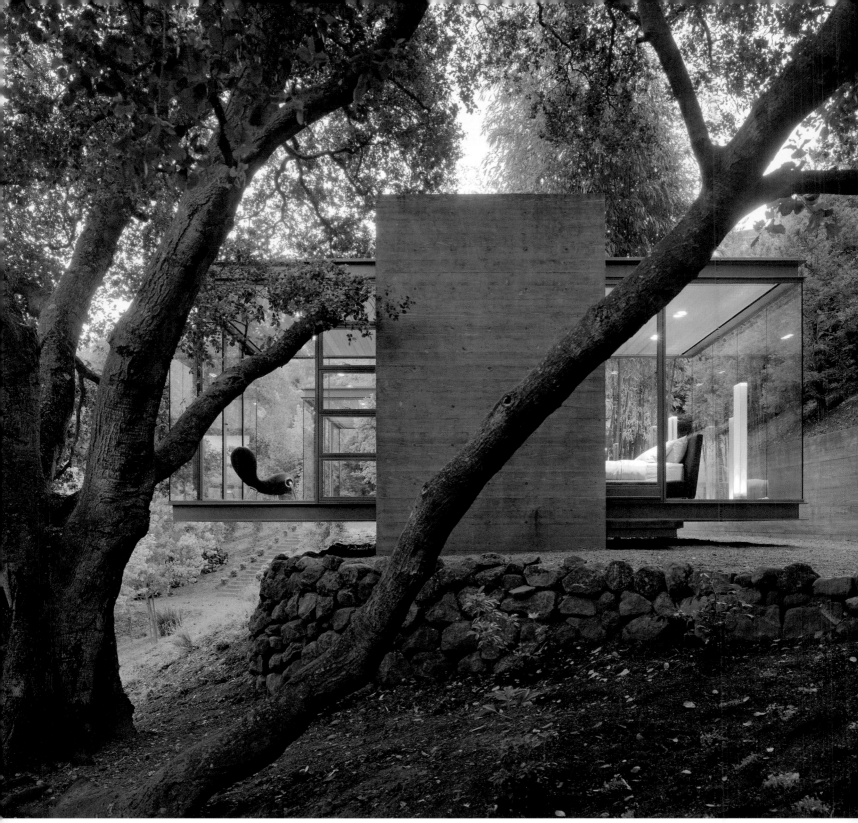

view from exterior

Tea Houses

Silicon Valley, USA

Architect: Swatt | Miers Architects
Location: Silicon Valley, California, USA
Year of completion: 2009
Area: 127 sqm
Type of retreat: tea houses

The idea for the tea houses originated when the client and architect partnered years ago to sustainably remodel the 6,000-square-foot main house. During construction the client found respite in a remote location on the site, below a ridge beneath a grove of Heritage California Live Oaks. The high-tech Silicon Valley executive wanted to create a place where he could simply withdraw into nature. Years later the vision was realized as three individual tea houses. The 270-square-foot "meditating" tea house, nestled under the canopy of the largest oak tree, is a place for individual meditation. The slightly larger "sleeping" tea house, approximately 372 square feet, is a space designed for overnight stays. At 492 square feet, the "visioning" tea house is for intimate gatherings and creative thinking.

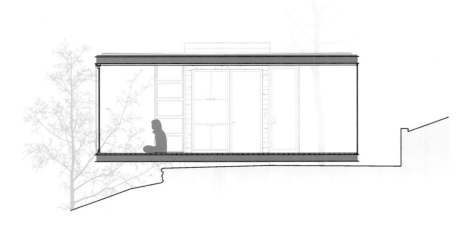

from above to below, from left to right: section, panorama view,
entrance, exterior view

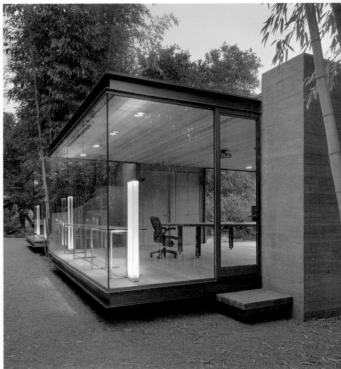

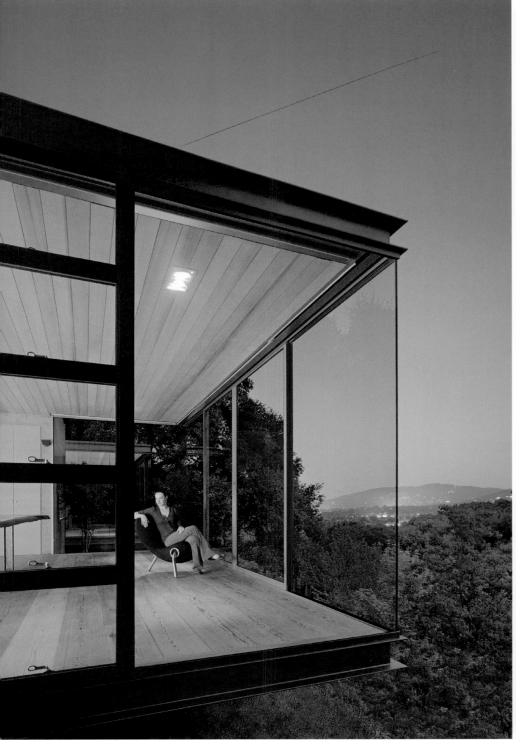

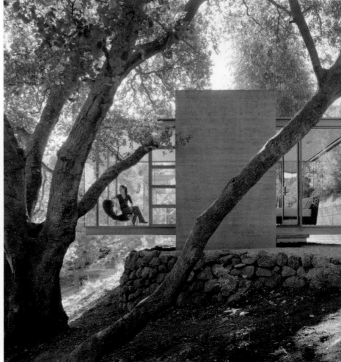

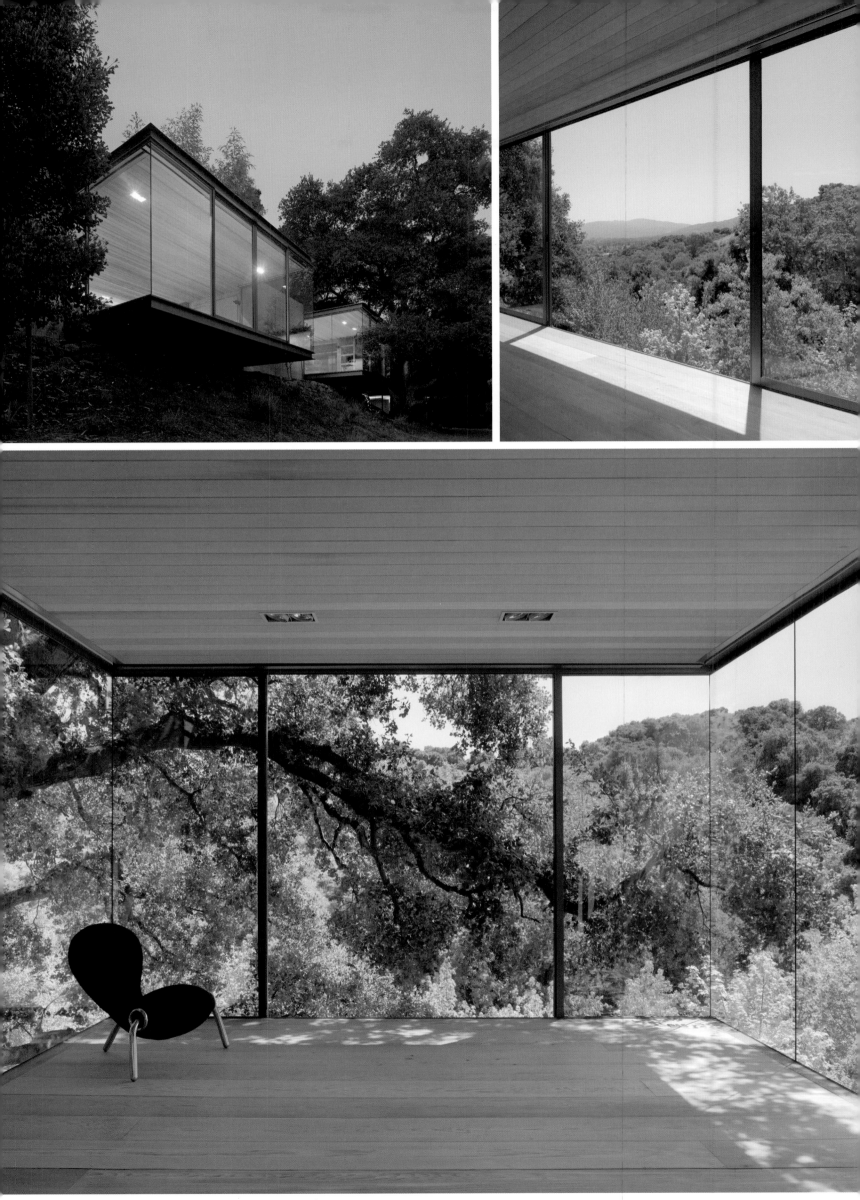

from left to right, from above to below: exterior view at night,
perspective, interior view

157

Index

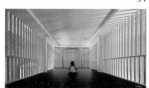
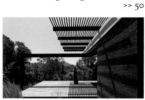
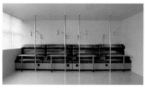
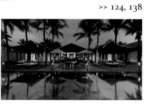
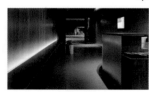
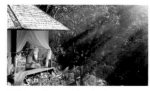
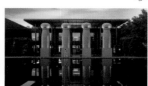
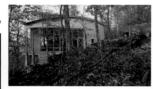
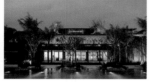
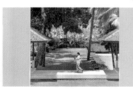
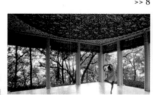
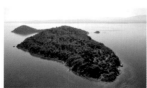
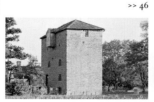
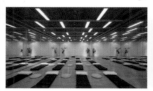
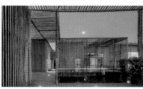
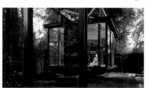
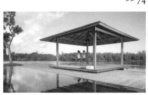
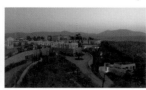
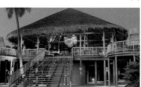
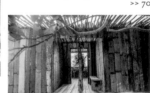
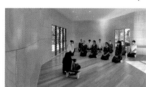
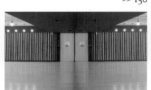
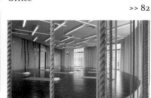
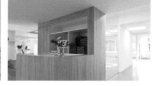
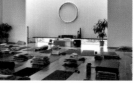
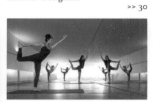
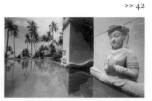
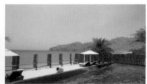
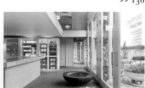
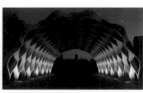
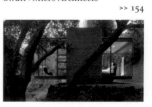

Tobias Partners

>> 14

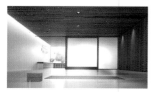

27 Renny Street, Paddington
NSW 2021 (Australia)
T +61 2 9361 4800
studio@tobiaspartners.com
www.tobiaspartners.com

Wendell Burnette Architects

>> 26

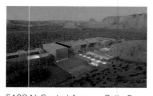

5102 N. Central Avenue, Suite 5
Phoenix, Arizona 85012 (USA)
T + 602 395 1091
F + 602 395 0839
info@wendellburnettearchitects.com
www.wendellburnettearchitects.com

Wimberly Allison Tong & Goo

>> 102

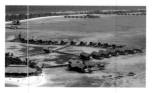

Boston House
36-38 Fitzroy Square
London, W1T 6EY (UK)
T +44 20 7906 6600
F +44 20 7906 6660
london@watg.com
www.watg.com

WMR Arquitectos

>> 66

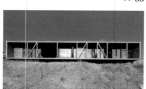

Centinela de Matanzas s/n 7a
Región 4066, Vitacura Espoz
(Chile)
T +97 44 24 39
info@wmrarq.cl
www.wmrarq.cl

Picture Credits

All other pictures were made available by the architects
and/or hotels.